gut insight

probiotics and prebiotics for digestive health and well-being

by Jo Ann Tatum Hattner, MPH RD
with Susan Anderes, MLIS

Suggested Cataloging
Hattner, Jo Ann Tatum.
Gut insight: Probiotics & prebiotics for digestive health and well-being
by Jo Ann Tatum Hattner, MPH, RD with Susan Anderes, MLIS.
123 pp. 28 cm.
1. Digestive organs — Popular works. 2. Bacteria — Health aspects.
3. Probiotics — Popular works. 4. Prebiotics — Popular works.
I. Anderes, Susan M. II. Title

ISBN-10 0-578-02615-2
ISBN-13 978-0-578-02615-2

QP145 H378 2009
612.3

Website: www.gutinsight.com

Dedicated to Mother Nature who is minding the microbes.

Disclaimer

This book is written for basically healthy people who want to improve their health. If you have any health issue, such as a chronic disease or an immune compromised condition, see your physician. The authors disclaim responsibility for any adverse affects that may result from the use of the information contained in this book.

Acknowledgements

We would like to extend our thanks to:

John Kerner, MD, Alan Lake, MD, and Jose Saavedra, MD, physicians who specialize in gastroenterology who so willingly shared their knowledge and expertise. We thank them for reviewing chapters, correcting our errors, and answering our questions.

Ann Coulston, nutritionist, Ashini Srivastava, physician, Marlene Lucas, nurse, Donna Hjertberg, technical writer, our initial reviewers and peers.

John Allan, MS for contributing information about the National Yogurt Association's "Live & Active Cultures" seal.

Michael DeAngelis, MS, MPH, RD for his assistance in interpreting the almond research.

Mary Ellen Sanders, PhD for her contributions and explanations.

Bryan Tungland, MS for generously sharing his expertise on inulin.

Mark Uebersax, PhD for educating us on the properties of beans.

Miguel Freitas, PhD and Juli Hermanson, MPH, RD for fact checking sections on their products.

To Elaine Kesey, Sheryl Kesey Thompson, Jennifer Giambroni, Liz Reinhiller Housman, Patama Roj, Danielle Madsen, Jennifer Lim, Marina Nikolenko, Velvet Gogol Bennett, and Sarah Badger who provided permissions and details about specific products containing probiotics and prebiotics.

Harold McGee for his book *On Food and Cooking*, our best resource on specific foods.

Lucille Sutton for her copyediting and guidance.

Most importantly we recognize all of the university affiliated researchers including Glen Gibson, Marcel Roberfroid, Alanna Moshfegh, Jan Van Loo, Allan Walker, Jose Saavadra, and Erika Isolauri, whose work contributed to the scientific basis for the book.

Contents

Introduction

The cure is within your body — the secret for wellness! You can restore what aging, stress and anxiety, lack of sleep, poor eating habits, exposure to infections, and illness have done to damage this natural process. Rather than take a bevy of pills, you can take better care of yourself and bolster your immune system. There is a natural way to bring internal health and enhanced immunity back. And it is not hard to do!

As a result of research linking probiotic use to enhanced immunity and digestive health, the marketplace floodgates have opened and consumer interest is surging. Meanwhile, food manufacturers are utilizing research to their advantage and are marketing a variety of foods enhanced with probiotics. As scientific articles promote their benefits and consumers ingest the products with positive health results, the word is spreading that the cure comes from inside you and it is within your reach.

As a nutritionist at Stanford University Medical Center and in private practice, I have counseled hundreds of patients with "digestive ills" and "bad stomachs" who have suffered chronic constipation, diarrhea, bloating, and gas. I've found that the addition of live cultures to their daily diets has had a remarkable effect on restoring their natural balance, and thus their health and comfort. Indeed, I am convinced that probiotic use in most people can enhance their immunity, promote regularity, lessen gas and bloating, and yes, even enhance their sex life!

Consider Josh, the hard-charging young businessman who came to me for nutritional counseling. Still only in his thirties, he was suffering from diarrhea, which made him fear his frequent business flights. Sometimes the urgency forced him to hastily leave a business meeting in search of a bathroom. Josh's doctor had recently put him on a lactose free diet suspecting that his diarrhea was due to his inability to digest lactose, a natural component of milk. But after a month on the lactose free regime, Josh was not feeling better.

As I learned more about Josh, his diet, and his lifestyle, I suspected that his digestive tract bacteria were out of balance. I first suggested using fermented foods, such as yogurt containing live active cultures, to correct the imbalance and alter the dynamics of his gut. But we both realized that with his hectic travel schedule this was not realistic. So we agreed that he would take a daily probiotic supplement — one specific strain that had been studied for the relief of irritable bowel syndrome. Since it was a supplement, Josh cleared it with his doctor. In about a month's time, with the use of the probiotic and some minor lifestyle changes to reduce stress, his symptoms began to improve. Six months later he sent a message via Blackberry that he was amazed that such a simple and natural remedy could make such a difference.

Ella, a housewife in her fifties, came to see me in exasperation over her chronic constipation. "I will be very up front. I have been constipated all of my life. I thought it was caused by tensions with my mother, but now my mother is gone and I am still suffering from constipation." On her initial visit she revealed that she had tried every available stool softener on the market and occasionally used laxatives. In addition, she had increased the fiber sources in her diet, including whole fresh fruits and salads, flax seed, and psyllium, but the added fiber was giving her gas often at the most embarrassing times, such as during yoga class.

Ella feared she was becoming dependent upon pharmaceutical remedies and came to me in search of more natural diet remedies. First we discussed the natural sources of fiber found in a wide variety of whole grains that she could easily add to her diet. We then explored other foods in her diet. Ella liked dairy products but tended to shy away from them as she believed they were constipating. I explained to her that not all dairy products are the same and pointed her to a yogurt product with live active cultures which had been shown to shorten intestinal "transit time", moving the stool through the bowel more rapidly than was normal for her. This was a product with the potential to provide the natural therapy she was seeking. Ella agreed to try it. She began aggressively, eating two cartons of the yogurt a day, but after a few weeks she was able to cut it to one a day with favorable results. She has achieved regularity.

Kelly, who is a college student and newly engaged to be married, came to me suffering from gas and bloating. To slim down, she had been trying various diets, including the cabbage soup diet and the cereal diet. Meanwhile her fiancé had given her a sexy Victoria's Secret nightgown. "But, I was so bloated and in pain with gas there was no way I was going to put it on, much less engage in any romantic activity."

What she wanted from me was advice on a weight loss diet without the bloating and gas. First, we discussed making some changes in her lifestyle to increase her physical activity. She agreed she could walk to class and hike with her fiancé. Then together we planned a calorie plan for weight loss that included a moderate amount of fiber. But I told her I really wanted her to bolster her digestive health by adding foods with natural cultures of probiotics. We chose soy-based foods because of her allergy to dairy foods.

Within four weeks, Kelly had lost just two pounds, however, her abdomen was flatter with less gas. It took her another six weeks to drop eight pounds. But now that she was without the gas and bloating, she had the courage to take the Victoria's Secret nightgown out of her drawer.

These clients, and now you, are learning of the healthful benefits of probiotics, which are natural cultures of beneficial bacteria. Once ingested, probiotics work their magic by traveling to sites in your gut, where they cultivate your beneficial bacteria and stimulate a healthy response. *Probiotic* originates from Greek with *pro* meaning promoting and *biotic* meaning life. They are present in naturally fermented foods such as yogurt and kefir. Or they can be taken in capsule form. The concept was first presented in 1908 when Dr. Ilya Mechnikov (sometimes spelled as Eli or Elie Metchnikoff), a Nobel Prize winning physician, correlated the longevity and health of Bulgarian peasants with a diet plentiful in foods fermented with a bacteria that he isolated and named *Lactobacillus bulgaricus*. Most importantly he recognized that bacteria was essential to health.

For many years probiotic therapy was used primarily by alternative medicine practitioners, but as a result of new research linking bacteria to immunity as well as health-driven consumers' increasing demand, probiotic use has become mainstream.

Why you should care?

Did you know that seventy percent of immune function takes place in your gut? It makes sense as this is where the body encounters the majority of pathogens. Think of your gut as your immune system's command center — responsible for the regulation of your responses, particularly of inflammation. Inflammation serves a protective role responding to tissue injury or infection so that you can heal. However, if you have chronic inflammation, it can lead to the development of disabling conditions such as inflammatory bowel disease, arthritis, atherosclerosis, or psoriasis. In numerous studies of all age groups, regular probiotic use enhances immunity. Enhanced immunity gives you the edge to perform better, have more energy, and stay healthy and positive.

Gut Insight will teach you about probiotics and prebiotics and how they can positively influence your health and well-being: what probiotics and prebiotics are, why they are necessary for gut health and immunity, which foods contain them, and how to integrate them into meals and snacks.

You will gain insight into how probiotics and prebiotics work together to create a healthy environment in your gut, which will in turn positively influence immunity and well-being. You will find resources for shopping emphasizing whole natural foods. You will learn about specialty probiotic foods and beverages. You will become skilled at preparing foods using ingredients that enhance probiotic effects with our recipes and resources.

Glossary

Bowel transit time The amount of time it takes for ingested food to travel through your GI tract and pass out as stool.

Gut Site of digestion, absorption, immune function, and elimination.

Lactose intolerance The inability to digest lactose, the natural sugar of milk. Symptoms may include bloating, gas, diarrhea, and discomfort.

Milk allergy Hypersensitivity to milk protein.

Pathogenic bacteria Disease causing bacteria which can cause both damage to the gut tissue and infections.

Prebiotics Nondigestible food ingredients that selectively stimulate the growth and/or the activity of beneficial bacteria in the colon and improve health.

Probiotics Live microorganisms which, when consumed in adequate amounts, confer a health benefit on the host.

Chapter One: Probiotics

Probiotics function in the gut to provide a health benefit.

What are Probiotics?

Probiotics are live microorganisms (mostly bacteria) which are so very tiny you can't see them. They provide beneficial effects in your gut by contending with injurious microorganisms and enhancing immunity. Because of the health benefits attributed to these beneficial bacteria, probiotics are added to common foods. This concept of adding probiotics to foods was given scientific credibility with an authoritative report on health and the nutritional properties of probiotics in food by the Food and Agricultural Organization of the United Nations and the World Health Organization in 2001. The report defined probiotics as "live microorganisms which, when consumed in adequate amounts, confer a health benefit on the host."

The addition of live microorganisms to foods is not a new concept as people have been doing it for hundreds of years. Many familiar foods which you may enjoy are made with live microorganisms. These include fermented dairy foods such as yogurt, kefir and cheeses, and other foods such as sour dough bread, dill pickles, sauerkraut, kim chi, tea, beer, and wine. The practice of adding live cultures of probiotic bacteria to foods to provide health benefits is very familiar in Asia and Europe, but is relatively new to the US. But as reported in the media adding probiotic bacteria to foods is "catching on like wildfire." Probiotic products are proliferating. New foods are added daily with the market driven by scientific findings connecting the benefits of probiotics to an enhanced immune response and digestive health. Probiotics added to yogurt products may already be familiar to you, however, as you will read and learn in this and future chapters there are numerous new foods with probiotics in dairy and soy products, in cereal, in energy bars, in specialty drinks, and in infant formula.

Advances in food technology provide processes which encapsulate, freeze dry, and dehydrate microorganisms. They can then be added to foods, survive storage, and be reactivated in the gut when ingested.

From a nutritional view, adding foods with probiotics to your diet, particularly foods which are originally made with live active organisms or starter cultures such as yogurt, kefir, and some cheeses, is preferred to taking supplements. The best course of action is to make eating healthy foods with live active cultures a lifelong habit. Probiotics in powder or capsule form (supplements) are useful treatment of a specific condition such as irritable bowel syndrome. Here we focus on food and beverage sources and recommend taking probiotic supplements only under a doctor's supervision.

Glossary

Terms often used interchangeably.

Microorganisms Microscopic living organisms.

Microbes Any minute form of life.

Bacteria Single cell microscopic living organisms with 500 – 1000 different species in the intestine alone.

Microflora Bacteria and other microorganisms that inhabit an area, (e.g., the intestinal tract).

Microbiota A term used by researchers to replace microflora.

Bacteria within Your Body

In order to understand the science behind the probiotic concept you do need to know a little bit about the inside of your body and what you are made of. Like it or not, as humans we are made up of a lot of things including bacteria — single cell living microorganisms. In fact, our bodies have ten times more microbial cells than the total number of other cells. The microorganisms (mostly bacteria) reside primarily in our gut where there are over 500 different types. In the gut they primarily perform necessary and beneficial functions — digestive and defensive roles such as providing protection against chronic inflammation and decreasing reactions to allergens as well as B vitamin synthesis. In addition, they safeguard the integrity of the cells that line the gut by inhibiting the growth of pathogenic bacteria. Pathogenic (disease causing) bacteria can also reside in our gut, and they can cause both damage to the gut tissue and infections, so it's important to keep the beneficial bacteria in the majority. You can do that by ingesting probiotics.

It All Started with Birth

You may be wondering where your resident bacteria originally came from. Before birth you were protected by amniotic fluid in the womb and had very little exposure to bacteria. With birth, the journey down the vaginal canal exposed you to your mother's bacteria and after birth, her touch, her kisses, her breast and her breast milk exposed you to more of your mother's bacteria. Your mother's gift was instrumental in the development of your own immune response and protected you from the hostile elements in the environment into which you were born. It provided a protective gut barrier and defense mechanisms to shield you from infectious diseases. As you grew, you were exposed to more bacteria and by about your second birthday, you developed an identifiable population of microorganisms in your gut known as your microbiota. Some researchers refer to this resident population as your microbiota fingerprint as they believe it is an individual pattern which defines you for a lifetime. Researchers theorize that both genetics and the environment contribute to the fingerprint's makeup.

Throughout life, the numbers will change and there will be modifications of bacterial types with pathogenic bacteria introduced by infections. Good bacteria can be wiped out by the use of antibiotics, poor diet, stress, or ingestion of pathogens in food, but basically your body tries to maintain its fingerprint. As you get older, the total population of microbiota decreases reducing the good bacteria and providing less protection from disease. Remember Dr. Ilya Mechnikov who identified and named the bacterium *Lactobacillus bulgaricus*? He correlated longevity with the regular ingestion of foods fermented with this bacterium.

Researchers in the fields of immunology, infectious disease, and basic science have been examining this microbial world that resides within us. They are progressing towards an understanding of microbes' role in the prevention and treatment of chronic conditions and diseases. Obesity has been the recipient of a great deal of research and researchers have now suggested that overweight people have different kinds of microbes in the gut than lean people. They recognize that this may be related to the breakdown and storage of food. The initial interpretation is that the obese person may have the ability to extract more calories from their food.

More discussion of research and benefits in particular conditions follow in future chapters. For now we summarize the benefits of probiotics currently described in the scientific literature as well as those under investigation.

Benefits described by scientists are:
- immunity enhancement
- improvement in lactose digestion
- management of diarrhea in infants
- treatment of constipation
- improved tolerance to antibiotic therapy
- reduced symptoms of respiratory infections

Benefits currently under investigation include:
- beneficial effects on cholesterol profiles
- prevention of diarrhea
- prevention of allergy in infants
- treating symptoms of irritable bowel syndrome
- treating inflammatory bowel disease — especially ulcerative colitis
- vaginal health
- beneficial effects on oral health.

New Research Directions

Papers documenting research on the use of probiotics to treat specific conditions or disease symptoms continue to appear. An important area of research is the prevention of colon cancer. Many disease protective processes involve an immune response, so research is conducted by immunology and infectious disease specialists, cancer specialists, and microbiologists. Scientists are working hard to unravel the mysteries of the microbiota and its role in our gut and overall health.

"Crosstalk" a New Buzzword

You may still be questioning why it's a good thing to eat foods with beneficial bacteria (probiotics). The obvious answer is that eating foods with probiotics will enhance the population of beneficial bacteria in your gut. Think of it this way: the gut houses a lot of bacteria in a complex ecosystem. This ecosystem is in direct communication with your immune system. Your immune system protects and preserves you and is responsible for your body's health. It starts protecting you in the epithelial lining of your mouth, continues to the stomach, the small intestine, and the colon.

Scientists have found that there is a complex relationship with the immune system, its response, and the microbiota. In fact they have even provided a new term to describe this relationship, it is "crosstalk." Crosstalk refers to the communication between the microbiota of your gut and your immune system. It involves interaction and coordination of not only the gut microbiota, but also of the cells lining the gut.

A Probiotic Journey

So you can have a better understanding of this concept, let's meet Brittany and take a probiotic journey[1]. Brittany, mother of two teenage boys and a second grade teacher, focuses on good health and well-being. She is continually in contact with people on the bus who are sneezing or coughing or in her classroom where her children share not only their recent experiences, but their colds and other illnesses. At home Brittany must meet the demands of a working mother. Brittany is characterized by her friends as "the one with the most energy and fastest walker." She lives a healthy lifestyle.

What is her secret? Brittany has found that if she keeps her immune system in good working order she is able to get through even the toughest of winters without respiratory illness, colds, or coughs. She begins her morning by rising earlier than anyone else in the household so she has time for breakfast. And on the days when she is rushed, she packs her breakfast to eat at school. Her typical breakfast is yogurt with live active cultures of a *bifidobacteria* (a probiotic), accompanied with some whole grain bread, muffin, or cereal.

---

[1] Reid R. So, which bacteria did you eat today? 2005, Danone Vitapole DVD video.

The moment the yogurt enters her mouth the *bifidobacteria* begin their work destroying pathogenic bacteria in her mouth, bacteria which can cause plaque buildup and inflammation of her gums. The *bifida* travel down her throat and esophagus to her stomach, protected by the fermented milk in the yogurt; they survive the acidic gastric juices of the stomach and reach her small and large intestine. In her intestine the *bifida* receive signals warning of the presence of dangerous pathogenic bacteria that have entered the gut either from the environment or from contaminated food sources. Armed with signaling devices, the *bifida* are theoretically able to coordinate with the immune modulating cells (essentially messengers) to deploy protective mechanisms, shielding Brittany's gut barrier from pathogens that can break across that barrier and cause illness or inflammation.

Because the *bifida* may also destroy the pathogens themselves, *bifida* are good bacteria for Brittany to cultivate. In Brittany's colon, *bifida* enjoy a meal of prebiotics which are nondigestible carbohydrates from the whole grain muffin. This results in the production of acid, making the environment uninhabitable for pathogenic bacteria which in turn results in their quick demise. The probiotic *bifida* continue their journey on through Brittany's colon and in a day or two end up as part of her poop (feces). Because the *bifida* do not stay around, it is recommended that they be ingested daily or every other day to continue to cultivate the good bacteria in the gut. Brittany is one of many who have discovered the advantages of eating foods with added probiotics for digestive health and enhanced immunity.

Microorganisms with probiotic status have been demonstrated to stimulate the immune system. These are primarily lactic acid bacteria, that is, bacteria that produce lactic acid in the gut. So, in addition to stimulating the immune system, they increase the acidity of the gut inhibiting the growth of undesirable bacteria. Yes, they inhibit the kind of undesirable bacteria that can make you sick.

The Probiotic Concept

Most of the bacteria that reside in our bodies are not harmful. The ones that are, however, can cause infections, such as infectious diarrhea, and they can produce byproducts that can be harmful to our gut and its environment. One way to counteract these destructive consequences is to cultivate probiotics. Probiotics contribute to a healthy balance of the gut microbiota. Yes, not only do you eat a "balanced diet" and enjoy a "balanced life" but now you also "balance your microbiota." Perhaps this is a new concept — one you never considered before. But you have most likely suffered from a bad episode of "food poisoning" or after traveling arrived home with not just your baggage but a bad case of "traveler's revenge", so you do have an inkling of the role of harmful bacteria. Using probiotics as a preventive or treatment therapy for these conditions is very appealing.

Probiotic Criteria

How do we know which bacteria are probiotics? Probiotics are distinctive microorganisms; they must meet the following criteria in order to be given probiotic status.

A probiotic:

- is a microbial organism which is not harmful (pathogenic)
- remains viable (alive) during processing and shelf life of the food
- must survive digestion and remain viable in the gut
- is able to bring about a response in the gut
- is associated with health benefits.

As with most things in science the criteria are continuing to develop.

Listing of Commonly Used Bacteria

The most commonly used sources of probiotics in food in the United States are various strains of *lactobacillus* and *bifidobacterium*. This is a listing of the genus and species within that genus. For example *Lactobacillus* is the genus and *acidophilus* is the species.

Common Probiotic Bacteria

- *Lactobacillus acidophilus*
- *Lactobacillus casei*
- *Lactobacillus reuteri*
- *Lactobacillus plantarum*
- *Lactobacillus rhamnosus*

- *Bifidobacterium animalis*
- *Bifidobacterium lactis*
- *Bifidobacterium infantis*
- *Bifidobacterium longum*

The entire species may not function within the probiotic concept. Specific strains within a species have been scientifically tested and confirmed as having a probiotic effect such as *L. Rhamnosus GG*. The *L.* is the genus (*Lactobacillus*), *rhamnosus* is the species and *GG* is the strain. This is just one in a listing of many strains which have been tested and are being used commercially. In addition, the yeast *Saccharomyces cerevisiae (boulardii)* is also used in foods such as kefir.

Conclusion

Probiotics need to survive the treacherous path through the stomach (where some bacteria are destroyed, both good and bad) and down the small intestine into the large intestine where they can do their job and carry on their natural healthful activities. Taking probiotics in foods actually helps to protect them during this journey by providing a protective shield against the acid in the stomach. Now we will discuss where to find these foods, how to read the labels, and how to evaluate their content.

Chapter Two: Probiotic Food Sources

Managing Your Gut Health with a Diet Rich in Probiotics.

You learned in chapter one that both beneficial and harmful microbes compete for positioning and housing in your gut and that protective microbes (probiotics) and illness provoking microbes are poised to do battle. Gut health depends upon which microbes win and remain in the majority. You also learned that you can influence the diversity and the majority of protective microbes by eating foods with probiotics. By strengthening the body's defenses you have the potential to protect yourself from a whole host of chronic illnesses.

As the food industry is fortifying foods to make them healthier and provide targeted benefits, expect to see more and more foods containing probiotics in the marketplace.

Searching for Probiotics in Foods

Reading labels on food packages can be overwhelming. To teach you about reading labels let's start with an example of one of the most popular probiotic containing foods: yogurt. The same criteria apply whether the yogurt is dairy or soy.

There are two important things to consider when scanning the carton:

First: Does it have live and active cultures?
        Easy to tell from the label.

Second: Do the cultures qualify as proven probiotics?
        Difficult to tell as manufacturers may not identify strains.

The cultures refer to the bacterial cultures and live means they are living or viable. They must be live to be of any benefit. The starter cultures used for fermentation of milk to make yogurt are commonly *Lactobacillus bulgaricus* and *Streptococcus thermophilus*, which are added to milk after pasteurization. Each culture encourages the growth of the other and together they rapidly acidify the milk, resulting in yogurt. The amount of live and active cultures that are in the yogurt when you buy it is important.

Live Active Culture Seal

The National Yogurt Association has made it easy for you to recognize some products with live and active cultures with the development of their seal as shown below.

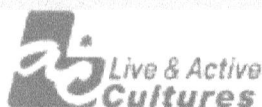

The National Yogurt Association (NYA) is the national non-profit trade organization representing the manufacturers and marketers of live and active culture yogurt products as well as suppliers to the yogurt industry. Its purpose is to sponsor health and medical research for yogurt with live and active cultures and serve as an information source to the trade and the general public. See: www.aboutyogurt.com

The helpful "Live & Active Cultures" seal assures that the product must contain at least 100 million combined *Lactobacillus bulgaricus* and *Streptococcus thermophilus* bacteria per gram of yogurt at the time it is made. These bacteria are considered to be probiotics as they provide a health benefit by relieving lactose intolerance. The seal does not provide any information on other cultures that may be present.

Importantly, when you see just the statement "live and active cultures," especially without the NYA seal, be aware that not all of the cultures are necessarily probiotics, even if the carton includes a statement that assures you that probiotics are in the ingredients. You have to just assume probiotic strains were used. Remember, there is no legal definition for the term probiotic, only a scientific definition that it is safe, viable, and when consumed in sufficient quantities, provides a health benefit.

One Yogurt Example

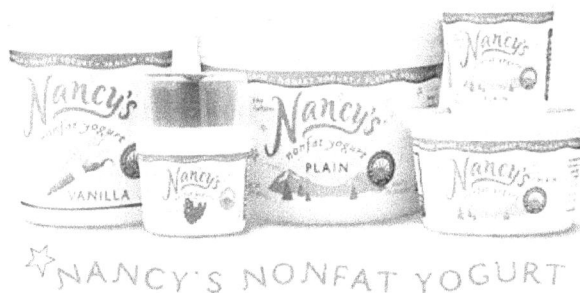

☆NANCY'S NONFAT YOGURT

However, not all yogurt manufacturers choose to use the live active cultures seal. Instead you may see a statement on the carton: "Live Cultures" with the specific cultures listed in the ingredients. You can check out their cultures by going to their web site. For example Springfield Creamery in Eugene, Oregon makes Nancy's cultured dairy yogurt — both conventional and organic — and soy yogurt which is all organic. They have one of the best and most educational websites www.nancysyogurt.com with knowledgeable people to answer your questions, if you should write to them. Note the ingredients: skim milk, nonfat dry milk powder, *L. acidophilus, S. thermophilus, L. bulgaricus, L. casei, L. rhamnosus, B. bifidum* cultures.

Elaine Kesey of Nancy's Yogurt responded by email to my question of specific strains with the following statement about the cultures they use to make Nancy's Cultured Dairy: "We do use different strains of bacteria cultures for specific products. We have multiple sources and multiple strains. For example, in our yogurts, we use 3 strains of *acidophilus*, 3 strains of *bifidum*, 3 strains of *casei* and 2 strains of *rhamnosus* — these strains from 3 different sources as well as one strain each of *bulgaricus* and *thermophilus*." Soy yogurt has similar, but non-dairy based bacterial cultures and promises "billions of live beneficial bacteria in each teaspoon of Nancy's just as it does for the dairy yogurt."

Informational Websites

For more information on any yogurt product, I advise you to investigate the manufacturer's web site for descriptions of their live cultures. In addition, you can contact the manufacturer directly and ask for the specific strains used and whether or not they have been studied. An excellent resource is the Questions and Answers section online at www.usprobiotics.org. Check out their section on Products with Probiotics.

Right now, no established legal definition for the term probiotic exists. US manufacturers of food and beverages can make the claim that a product contains "probiotics" providing specific benefits without meeting any Food and Drug Administration criteria. Many scientists, including Dr. Mary Ellen Sanders, a food microbiologist, have advocated that the manufacturers of food and beverages should meet criteria based on FAO/WHO guidelines.

Recommended labeling guidelines:

- the genus, species and strain of all microbes contained

- the count of live microbes at the end of the shelf life

- proper storage guidelines

- benefits based on human studies

- recommended levels of consumption

- a method for reporting any adverse effects.

Product Categories

The dairy case is bursting with products with live cultures. Besides the cartons of yogurt, there are drinkable kefir and smoothies — conventional and organic, dairy and soy. Here are a few product categories you can look for in the dairy case. There are national as well as regional brands. Remember in order to know if the product contains live cultures, check the container label for the live active culture seal or for the live active cultures in the ingredients. A recommended serving each day is between 4-8 ounces. You will adjust this as you find out what works for you.

Dairy Products

Yogurt in a carton

Yogurt is milk which has been fermented by bacteria into a tart thick semisolid mass.

Plain (non-fat yogurt, low-fat yogurt and whole milk yogurt)

Flavored, Fruit Blends, Light, Fruit on top

Greek style

Note: Most cup yogurts contain live active cultures, but there are exceptions — check the label.

Organic cup yogurt: Made from organic ingredients. Look for the USDA organic seal on the carton.

Cup yogurts contain a sell-by or buy-by date on the carton. Generally they must be used within 7-10 days after opening the carton. If the carton is unopened it is still safe to use within 7 days after the date, however, the live active culture counts may be lower than when the yogurt was fresher.

Specialty yogurts

Dannon™ Activia® for regularity, plain, Regular and Light flavored

Dannon™ DanActive® for enhanced immunity plain and flavored

Yoplait Yo-Plus™ for regulating digestive health

Use by the sell or buy date on the carton.

Smoothies

Flavored drinkable dairy yogurts both regular and light varieties.

Have a use by date. Drink them by that date for the best quality.

Kefir

A tart and effervescent fermented milk drink

Plain (unsweetened) and flavored

Organic

Other cultured dairy products

Yakult®, a cultured dairy drink that contains a proprietary bacterial strain, *Lactobacillus casei Shirota*.

Soy Products

Soy yogurt in a carton	Soybean milk which has been fermented by bacteria. Available in plain or flavored.
	Organic Look for "made with organic fruit and soy" or check the ingredients for organic ingredients, plain or flavored. (Note: because water is added to the soybeans to make the soymilk it does not qualify for the USDA organic seal).
Probiotic soy milk	Plain or flavored drinkable soy milk
Kefir	Made with soy milk and the same cultures as found in dairy kefir.

Greek Yogurt

Eating yogurt in the Mediterranean is such a different experience. Yogurt in Greece, for example, has a richer consistency and creamier taste than US yogurt. True Greek yogurt is strained and made from goats' milk. In the US, however, Greek yogurt is made from cows milk. It is ideal as a side dish complementing many foods. Greek yogurt is higher in protein and lower in carbohydrates than typical American yogurt. It is also higher in fat. So if you are watching your fat intake, you may want to try Oikos Organic Greek yogurt made by Stonyfield Farm. It has 0% fat and only 90 calories per 5.3 ounce serving. It is available plain or flavored with honey, vanilla, or blueberry.

The same starter cultures (*L. bulgararicus* and *S. thermophilus)* in conventional yogurt are used to make Greek style yogurts. You just have to be sure they are added after the milk is pasteurized, so they are still live. Stonyfield Farm adds three additional live probiotic cultures to Oikos Organic: *L. Acidophilus, Bifidus, and L. Casei*.

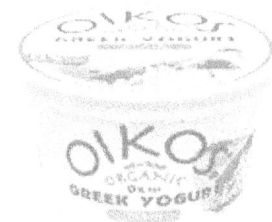

Kefir

Kefir, a cultured milk, is relatively new to the US marketplace. Although available since the 1970s in specialty stores, you can now find kefir in the dairy case in most stores. Unlike other fermented milks (yogurt, sour cream, buttermilk) kefir can be made with a unique process which incorporates kefir grains — large molecules which house as many as a dozen microbes including *lactobacilli*, *lactococci*, and yeasts. Manufacturers prepare kefir from a variety of starter cultures that they then list as ingredients on their label. Kefir has a creamy texture, a tart taste, and occasional effervescence. It makes great smoothies with a variety of juices. More recent additions to the market offer a variety of flavored kefirs.

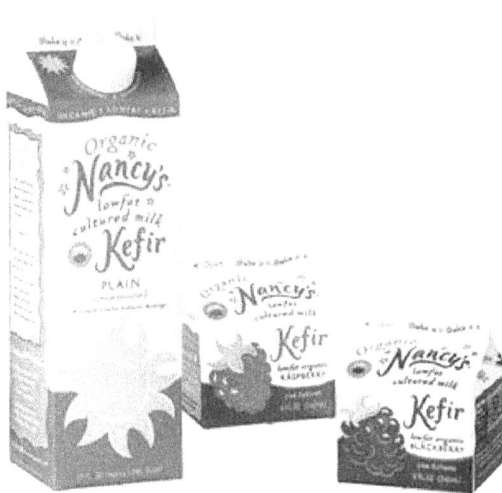

NANCY'S KEFIR

Kefirs do not have a seal like the yogurt manufacturers for live bacterial count. However, if you contact the manufacturer they may share their live microbial count per serving. Lifeway Foods makes the largest variety of kefir products — including conventional and organic dairy kefir, a nonfat dairy kefir, and organic soy kefir. The same ten starters are used for all. Lifeway reports that they offer about 7-10 billion CFUs per 8 ounces. The CFUs, colony forming units, are a measure of the count of bacteria, meaning they are capable of dividing and forming units of microbes. What you need each day will be very individual.

Because kefirs are a fermented product offering a variety of probiotics, think about incorporating them into your regular routine as a beverage or snack. Here are examples of Lifeway Foods (www.lifeway.net) products. They also make soy kefir and specialized kid-friendly kefirs in a pouch. The 10 starter cultures are the same for all their kefirs: *L. casei, L. acidophilus, L. plantarum, L. rhamnosus, B. bacterium breve, B. bacterium longum, S. diacetylactis, S. florentinus, S. lactis, Leuconostoc cremoris.*

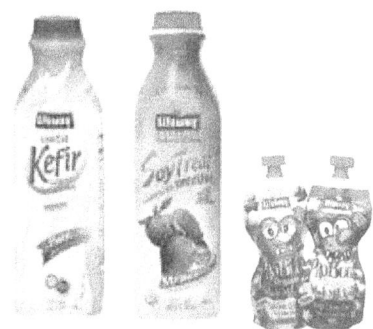

Cultured Dairy Drink

Yakult, a probiotic dairy drink, is now available in the US. It was developed in Japan over 70 years ago by microbiologist Dr. Minoru Shirota. Yakult assures that each 2.7 ounce bottle contains around 8 billion live and active *L. casei Shirota*, a proprietary probiotic strain exclusive to Yakult products. Numerous studies support the potential health benefits of Yakult. Drinking Yakult daily may help balance the digestive system, boost natural defenses, maintain regularity, and increase the amount of "good bacteria" in the digestive system.

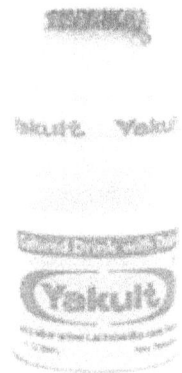

Soy Yogurt

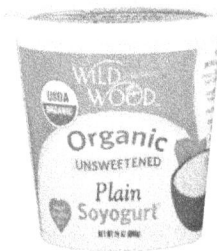

Soy yogurt is ideal for those of you who prefer soy to dairy. As yet there is no comparable live active culture seal for soy yogurt, so look for "active cultures" in the ingredients listing. Below is Wildwood Plain Yogurt carton. Wildwood™ states "Probiotic Cultures" on its carton but without the strains, only the genus and species of the active cultures in the ingredients listing. Wildwood ingredients list states: … Active Cultures (*S. Thermophilus, L. Bulgaricus, L. Acidophilus, L. Casei, L. Rhamnosus, B. Bifidum, L. Lactis*).

Try any of these products for at least two to three weeks and evaluate it for yourself. Fermented foods like yogurt and kefir have been associated with well-being for hundreds of years. So feel confident that you are enjoying a healthy food.

A Note about Frozen Yogurt

There is a revival of frozen yogurt shops which now offer frozen yogurt with live active cultures as well as "pro-yo" products appearing in the freezer section of the supermarket. Dairy science research shows that it is possible for the cultures to survive in a frozen product. However, it appears to be dependent upon the manufacturing method, the ingredients, and the strains that are used. You can check with the manufacturer or ask the store management to provide you with the science that shows their product provides live active cultures when you eat it.

What You Can Expect

Once you adopt the daily practice of eating foods with live cultures, you will notice changes within your body. The most obvious change is usually with bowel regularity. Your body is responding in a regular manner and you suffer less from gas, bloating, constipation, and diarrhea. All of this is reflective of a calmer gut. A calmer gut can change your whole persona: you feel better, you look better, and you have more social confidence. Those with lactose intolerance (the inability to digest lactose, the natural sugar of milk) will discover yogurt with live active cultures is usually well tolerated. The process of fermentation and the live cultures in the yogurt naturally digest lactose, so you are getting less lactose. Although yogurt and kefir are not magical foods, they are close!

Specialty Products with Specific Benefits

Strains of probiotics are not equal when it comes to health benefits. Health benefits are generally strain specific. You may have different individual needs from those of your friends or family members. Many of the possible effects are still being studied and although not definitively proven, there is a long list of potential health benefits suggested by research associated with particular strains. Consider experimenting with which yogurt brands work best for you.

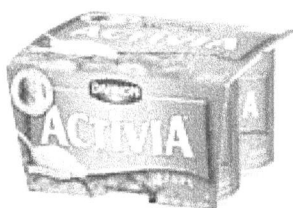
© Dannon Reprinted with Permission

Try different brands making sure they contain active probiotic cultures and see how you react and feel. Some combinations of strains have been studied and trademarked by yogurt manufacturers. Dannon has very thoughtfully designed a combination of active cultures which includes a proprietary probiotic strain *B. animalis DN 173 010 Bifidus Regularis*™. The ingredients list includes active cultures: *L. Bulgaricus, S. Thermophilus,* and *Bifidobacterium*.

Activia™ does help regulate the digestive system by helping with slow intestinal transit which is the time it takes the stool to pass through the lower bowel. But you need to eat it while the cultures are still active, so you want to always check the stamped date when you purchase it. In order for Activia™ to be effective it may require daily ingestion. Some people need 4 ounces or more, while others can use less daily and still experience the beneficial effects.

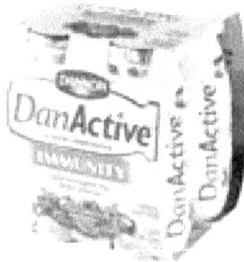

DanActive™ manufactured by Dannon™ contains trademarked *L. Casei Immunitas*™ cultures (*Lactobacillus casei* DN-114 001). The label reads "Contains the active cultures *L. Bulgaricus, S. Thermophilus* and *L. Casei Immunitas*™ The claim on the label reads: "Helps Strengthens your Body's Defenses. Probiotic Dairy Drink."

© Dannon Reprinted with Permission

Dannon™ has a collection of 25 scientific studies in humans, animals and in vitro (meaning in the lab not in a living organism) to support this claim. Their studies include results for these specific groups: children suffering diarrhea where the use of the product resulted in decreased diarrhea, students under stress taking exams where there was a demonstration of increased production of defense cells, seniors where there was a reduction of winter infections, and athletes showed a possible improvement in their defense response. You can review information on their website: www.danactive.com/danactive_scientific.html Each bottle of DanActive (3.3 fl ounces) contains 10 billion live and active *L. casei Immunitas*™ cultures (*L. casei strain DN-114 001*) that can survive and remain active in the digestive tract.

Other Foods with Probiotics

Cereals

Some cereals now contain probiotics. For example, Kashi The Seven Whole Grain Company™ has a cereal for digestive health with probiotics. It was the "first self-stable probiotic food." Their philosophy emphasizes their belief that "good digestive health puts you on the path to your best life." The manufacturer reports the strain used in the cereal as *L. casei*: *Lactobacillus paracasei ssp paracasei F19*. At the time of production, the cereal contains 1 billion *Lactobacillus casei* probiotic bacteria which are housed in the vanilla crisps. The cereal also contains ginger for digestive health.

Dry cereal may contain porbiotics in an encapsulated coating that becomes live and active once you eat the product. Select products that are labeled with descriptive viability statements such as: viable through the end of shelf life.

Wellness Bars

Bars are entering the market containing probiotics and are no longer referred to as energy bars. Rather they have new category names such as: probiotic wellness bars. Attune™ bars, available in the refrigerated dairy case of retailers throughout the US and online at www.attunefoods.com, contain probiotics that are specially formulated trademarked *LAFTI®* strains. The three strains contained are *L. acidophilus (LAFTI® L10), L. casei (LAFTI® L26), and B. lactis (LAFTI® B94)*. You will find these probiotic strains listed in the ingredients. Attune™ daily probiotic wellness bars come in two varieties and 10 flavors. The 100 calorie chocolate version (80 calories for dark chocolate), has a light, crunchy texture and the 170 calorie granola version, combines whole grains, nuts and dried fruit with a light yogurt-flavored coating. Attune bars are portable for daily use and are great for travel – the company states that the probiotics are good for 2-3 weeks at normal ambient temperatures.

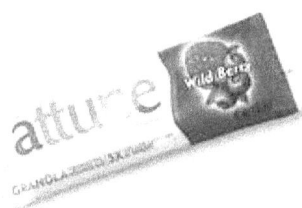

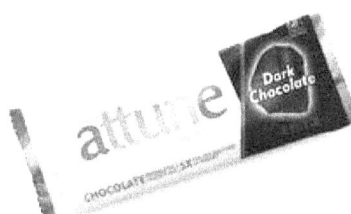

Savvy Consumption

Enhancing your total health by eating foods with probiotics requires that you also examine the total food and what it contributes to your diet. These foods can contribute not only probiotics, but high quality proteins, calcium, sodium, and potassium. You are the best judge of your own tolerance and the effectiveness of the product.

Dry products (cereals, bars) are digestive health foods. Unless the manufacturer assures you that you are getting adequate amounts of live active cultures of probiotics, you should consider them complementary rather than major sources of probiotics. Look for other components of those foods (protein content, fiber content, whole grains, dried fruits, total fat) before making your selection. The food may meet your criteria for a healthy food addition.

Conclusion

Developing the healthy habit of enhancing your gut health and immunity through the daily ingestion of healthy foods with probiotics is one thing you can do for yourself. Making probiotics a daily habit can enhance your health for a lifetime.

This chapter introduced you to foods with probiotics. In chapter three you will learn about prebiotics and their synergy with probiotics.

Glossary

Kefir A cultured milk made from a variety of starter cultures.

Specialty yogurts Yogurts marketed with claims of specific health benefits often associated with a proprietary bacterial strain.

Chapter Three: Prebiotics

Prebiotics are the booster substance for probiotics.

How Prebiotics Function

The complement to probiotics is prebiotics. In order to understand this concept let's look at how prebiotics function in your gut.

Interestingly, human milk contains small oligosaccharides that are undigestible by newborns. The role of these oligosaccharides in human milk was not at first understood and, in fact, researchers questioned why human milk would contain components unusable by the newborn infant. Scientists provided the explanation when they found that these small oligosaccharides were fueling beneficial *bifidobacteria* found in the newborn's gut. This explains why *bifidobacteria* is the predominant bacteria found in breast-fed babies.

Think of human milk as the original synbiotic food containing both probiotic bacteria and prebiotic carbohydrates to fuel bacterial growth. The prebiotic oligosaccharides in human milk are specific to human milk. However, this model has provided the stimulation and interest of food scientists for adding oligosaccharides to foods and beverages to enhance the growth of beneficial *bifidobacteria*.

When we eat a snack or a meal, acids and enzymes secreted in our stomach and small intestine digest our food releasing energy and nutrients that are absorbed and utilized by our bodies. But did you know that there are also nondigestible components in food that are primarily plant fibers? In plants, fibers or nondigestible carbohydrates have numerous functions, such as forming the cell wall which gives integrity to the plant. Consider, for example, celery, where you can see the fibers supporting the stalks. Fibers in plants are resistant to digestive acids and enzymes in your stomach and small bowel. They pass through the upper part of the gut undigested and when they reach the lower part of the gut — the colon — they are still whole. That is why when trying to lower calories in your daily diet, you are advised to increase your intake of plant foods — particularly high fiber vegetables. So you begin chomping on carrot and celery sticks, which fill you up, yet are not fully digested, so you absorb fewer calories. When the nondigestible carbohydrates reach the colon, enzymes produced by the microbiota can digest the fibers to yield fuel and nutrients necessary for their survival.

Glossary

Oligosaccharide Nondigestible fermentable carbohydrate.

Fructooligossacharide (FOS) A naturally occurring fructan sugar which acts like a fiber, passing undigested to the large intestine where it is extensively fermented by colonic bacteria.

The Prebiotic Approach

The prebiotic approach uses food with these nondigestible carbohydrates to stimulate growth and promote activity in beneficial microbiota. As the beneficial microbiota increases in number, pathogenic bacteria like *Salmonella*, *Campylobacter*, and *E. coli* decrease. This is a win-win situation for your gut health and for you.

Ingesting prebiotics is a practical way of manipulating your microbiota since they support and increase the probiotic population. Together they are an important duo. In addition, prebiotics are components of the healthiest foods on the planet — natural plant foods. That is why the whole grain muffin full of prebiotics was an excellent choice to accompany the yogurt in Brittany's breakfast as discussed in an earlier chapter.

When the nondigestible carbohydrates from the plant foods reach the lower bowel untouched by passage down the upper bowel, the microbiota go into action. This process, which results in the production of acids and gases, is fermentation. And yes, it takes place in your gut. However, there are numerous benefits.

Benefits of Fermentation for Your Gut and You

- **acids decrease the pH level (a measure of acidity and alkalinity)** of the colon. The lowered pH < 5.0 (acid milieu) is detrimental to the survival of disease causing bacteria.

- **short-chained fatty acid production** enhances the beneficial bacteria because the SFAs are their preferred energy source. In addition, they are used for energy by the cells lining the colon. Researchers are investigating a link between this function and the potential for suppressing cancer cell growth in the colon, suggesting that ingesting prebiotics affects the process of cancer production. Diets containing high concentrations of dietary fiber (nondigestible carbohydrates) and low concentrations of animal proteins and fat have been associated with reduced risks of colon cancer.

- **enhanced mineral absorption** — fermentation of the nondigestible fibers, particularly inulin from chicory root, enhances mineral absorption in the colon, especially calcium and magnesium. The change in acidity, as well as the production of short chain fatty acids, encourages this process. Studies have demonstrated this positive correlation in adolescent girls and post-menopausal women. You will see the claim "Inulin Boosts Calcium Absorption" on some foods that have inulin added as an ingredient, such as yogurt.

- **cholesterol lowering** — this effect is still being investigated with promising results in animal studies.

- **stabilizing blood glucose levels** — there are numerous studies investigating the potential effects of nondigestible fibers on regulating blood glucose levels and insulin response.

- **enhancing immunity** — beneficial gut microflora interact and communicate with cells lining the gut resulting in a positive immune response.

Downside of Fermentation

The single downside when you eat prebiotics is increased gas or flatulence. Gas results from the fermentation of fibers in the colon. You will notice increased gas production as you begin to increase plant sources. It is well known that vegetarians produce more gas, so perhaps we should consider gas a healthful sign. It's just gas. Passing gas ten to twenty times a day is normal for the average adult. You can alter your frequency of gas production by changing your diet. Although plant foods do produce gas, they are the healthiest foods, so look for other gas producing culprits to remove from your diet (for example, carbonated beverages).

Introducing more plant foods to your diet requires that you adopt the new diet slowly to allow your gut to adapt. Gas production varies with the total amount of fermentable foods ingested on a daily basis and also varies from person to person. Some people may experience discomfort which is a sign you should back off and eat less of those foods.

Scientific Criteria for Prebiotics

Just as there are lots of different bacteria but only a few designated as probiotics, there are relatively few designated prebiotics. Scientists have developed criteria for a substance to qualify as a prebiotic. Establishing criteria encourages research and identification of substances in foods which promote the growth of probiotics.

Professor Glenn Gibson of the University of Reading Food Biosciences Department in the UK and Marcel Roberfroid of the Université Catholique de Louvain in Brussels, Belgium coined the word "prebiotics" and developed criteria for a food substance to qualify as a prebiotic. A prebiotic food substance must:

- be nondigestible by the upper part of the gut.
- be utilized by beneficial microflora in the colon.
- result in selectively altering the microflora in the colon to a healthier composition.
- induce effects that are beneficial.

Based on these criteria, scientists and food manufacturers are isolating these substances and introducing them to foods — for example, inulin is added to yogurt, pasta, cereals, and cheeses. Natural food sources of prebiotics have been part of the human diet for centuries. We recommend that natural plant foods be part of your daily diet.

Prebiotic "Stars" and Prebiotic Potentials

Although all plant foods have nondigestible carbohydrates, not all plant foods have been studied and tested to determine if they are sources of prebiotics. The table below includes plant foods we consider to be prebiotic "stars" since they are the foods listed in the scientific literature as sources of prebiotics. We consider them to have a standing above other foods in importance. They contain the nondigestible carbohydrates that the probiotics need in order to thrive. We consider the foods in the list below without a star designation as **prebiotic potentials** meaning there are studies suggesting they may have a prebiotic effect, but they need more research, particularly human studies, to reach prebiotic status.

Prebiotic Stars* and Prebiotic Potentials

Fruits	apple, **banana***, berries, raisins
Vegetables	**onion***, **garlic***, **leeks***, **Jerusalem artichoke***, **globe artichoke***, **asparagus***, **chicory root***, **burdock***, **yacon***, jicama, tomato, greens: spinach, collard greens, chard, kale, mustard greens, **dandelion greens***, **salsify***
Legumes or pulses	legumes such as lentils, dry beans, chick peas and peas
Whole grains	**whole wheat***, **barley*** and **rye***, oats, brown rice, whole grain corn, buckwheat
Seeds	flaxseed, almonds
Other foods	honey

* These foods have been documented in the scientific literature as sources of inulin and oligosaccharides (nondigestible fermentable carbohydrates).

Just as with probiotics, scientists do not have a complete list. Most likely there are many, many more foods to be added as **prebiotic stars**. In the meantime it is wise to eat a wide variety of whole plant foods.

The Plant-Based Diet

Because the choices of prebiotics are all within plant food sources, let's review what a plant-based diet is. It is a diet based on eating foods that originate from plants.

That means you select and eat whole grains, vegetables, and fruits. In addition, you include beans and peas, nuts and seeds, and the oils that have a plant food source, for example olive oil or canola oil. You may also have dairy products, meat, poultry and fish in your diet, however, the majority of the foods are plant-based foods which offer calorie control, blood glucose control, and protection from the onset of chronic illnesses. There are volumes of scientific writings on the benefits of plant foods and the plant-based diet in the reduction of chronic illnesses such as heart disease, high blood pressure, and diabetes. And now you learn that plant foods are also the source of prebiotics. Really it should not be a surprise. If you believe in the "wholeness" of the body and the relationship of one bodily function to another, then it makes sense that the foods that are healthy for us also contribute to the health of our gut.

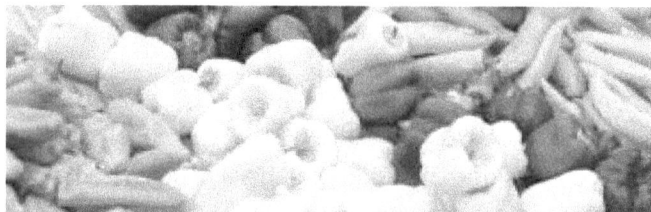

What about weight gain?

Some of you may be thinking as you are adding these new foods that you might gain weight — something you may not want to do. The best news is that adding plant foods to your diet will likely reduce your calories rather than increase them. Whole grains, fruits and vegetables, beans and peas are not really calorie laden and should most likely decrease your caloric intake.

But you may still be questioning whether dense foods like nuts might add calories. Well, almonds, for example, are 12 percent fiber — much higher than many of the other whole foods. Clinical studies have demonstrated that significant weight gain does not occur when almonds are substituted for other snacks as long as the portion size is reasonable. Studies have shown that the fat content of the almond is surrounded and encapsulated by cell walls which are not degraded in the upper part of the GI tract. This results in limited fat digestion and if you don't digest fat you don't acquire the calories.

In addition, a research study published in 2008 found that finely ground almonds significantly increased the levels of certain beneficial gut bacteria, thus concluding that the almond may have a prebiotic potential. Interestingly, this was demonstrated only with the ground almonds that contained the fat. When defatted almonds were used the beneficial bacteria growth was not demonstrated.

Benefits of Natural Plant Foods

Plants are full of phytochemicals (plant chemicals), which not only protect the plant from the onslaught of predators, such as insects, fungus and molds, but also protect you. For example, antioxidants protect your body cells from the naturally occurring ravaging free radicals believed to be responsible for the aging process. You can recognize phytochemicals in plants by their rich colors. An orange has 170 identified phytochemicals. Think of the rich color in tomatoes, lemons, peppers, strawberries, cherries, plums, and grapes to name just a few. The pigment is an indicator of its protective phytochemical content. Imagine when you eat a plant-based diet that you have an army of "internal defenders" protecting you.

Because people question whether they will get enough protein when they adopt a plant-based diet, we have selected some plant sources of protein for more in-depth discussion.

Pulses

There is one group of foods that is essential to include when adopting the plant-based diet. Does the name "pulses" ring a bell? It is a less familiar term for the plants of the legume family which includes peas, beans, lentils and chickpeas (garbanzos). Why should you include them? As you adopt the plant-based diet, you need to ensure adequate protein sources. You can do that by eating beans, lentils, and peas regularly.

Cultures all over the world use beans and lentils as the staple of their diet. Pulses provide fuel and protein, and are a rich source of the B vitamin folate. Beans and peas are lower glycemic index foods meaning they are beneficial for maintaining healthy blood glucose and insulin levels. The protein content of pulses complements the protein in grains so you get a full complement of amino acids (protein building blocks) by combining the two. In addition, here is your opportunity to use whole grains. Grains served with beans or lentils are traditional as main dishes throughout the world. You can begin to substitute some of your animal protein dishes with bean or lentil dishes using recipes that you will be able to find on our website: www.gutinsight.com.

Pulses don't have a great profit margin for grocers, so you may have to search for them. The supermarket staff typically shelves the beans and peas near the floor in a hard-to-find spot. The friendly market employee may not know the term pulses, so ask for dried beans or lentils. But remember, you can also find beans on the canned goods shelf. They are easy to use. Just open a can to use as a side dish or add to soups, stews, and salads!

Soy

The soybean has twice the protein of other legumes. The bean provides such a complete array of amino acids that its protein quality is similar to animal protein. For vegans, soy is essential, and for the rest of us, it is really very easy to include a variety of soy foods. One of the advantages of substituting soy for animal protein, for example meat, is that it doesn't contain the saturated fats, so it's healthier for your cardiovascular system. Soy foods are sources of phytochemicals including isoflavones which act as antioxidants. Foods that contain most of the bean are higher in isoflavone content — these include soy milk, sprouts, flour and tofu.

The bean is well known for its gas producing oligosaccharides. However, fermentation and other processing methods used to prepare soy foods result in products containing less of the gas producing substance. So the "gas" problem is really nothing to worry about, especially if you do as previously advised with any new plant food and add it in small amounts, increasing gradually.

Soy products at the market:

- **Bean curd or tofu** A concentrated mass of protein and oil made from soymilk. Originating in China where it was called Teu Fu, it is traditionally coagulated with calcium sulfate. The soft or silken tofu is full of moisture with a more delicate flavor. It is a delicious and easy to add to vegetable stir-fries, soups, and salads.

- **Fermented soy products** Tempeh, natto, soy sauce, and miso are all fermented soy products resulting from the microorganisms breaking down the protein, oligosaccharides, and other components into savory substances. Soy sauce has become a staple for flavoring and marinating, while miso is often used as a soup or a hot beverage made by stirring a little miso paste into hot water.

- **Edamame** These are immature soy beans so they are greener and sweeter. You can find them frozen, just boil for a few minutes in salted water and they are ready to eat as a snack or add to salads.

- **Soymilk** Made from the whole soybean now fortified with calcium and vitamin D is a substitute for cow's milk.

- **Soy yogurt** Made from soymilk and often with live cultures. It can be a source of probiotics; look for "live active cultures" on the label.

Plant-based Beverages – Tea and Coffee

Remember that your choice of beverage can be a plant-based beverage.

Tea is a beverage that has been used for its medicinal benefits for centuries. Somehow our ancestors figured out that tea is good "for whatever ails you." We know that tea is rich in certain compounds (polyphenols and phenolics) that have antioxidant powers. Antioxidants do just what their name implies; they protect the body's cells from the ravages of oxidation. Oxygen is good in your lungs, but it's not so great when it's floating around in your cells. The polyphenols in tea are not completely absorbed from the gastrointestinal tract and they too act just like the nondigestible carbohydrates and are utilized by the microbiota.

Let's look at just one study so you will understand tea's potential. A 2006 research project reported in Research in Microbiology looked at the effects of 31 different phenols extracted from tea on 28 different bacteria strains. Some of the bacteria were pathogenic, some normal, and some probiotic. The cultured cells were grown in dishes with the phenols. The findings demonstrated that the growth of the pathogenic bacteria was strongly inhibited, yet the growth of the probiotic bacteria were less affected. The scientists concluded that the growth of pathogenic bacteria may well be slowed down in the intestine while the probiotics would continue to grow and colonize. This study needs to be replicated, but meanwhile, try a self-treatment for your gut health with a cup of green or black tea. Yes, it needs to be green or black tea, since those two are the types with high polyphenol content. Decaffeinated is fine. Sit back and enjoy your morning "booster" while you get ready to take care of the day's business.

Coffee contains soluble fiber with phytochemicals — polyphenols and phenolics. Findings published in the Journal of Agricultural and Food Chemistry by scientists in Madrid reported that coffee (espresso, filtered or freeze dried) contains a significant amount of soluble dietary fiber and this dietary fiber contains a large amount of associated antioxidant phenolics. Studies such as those done with tea showing potential positive gut health effects need to be done with coffee.

Add a Little Chicory

Specialty coffees in New Orleans, the Caribbean, and Europe may contain chicory. Unfamiliar with chicory? Well, you would remember the bitter taste if you've tried it. One distributor of chicory (L' Epicerie) states "it is light and soothing on your stomach — brings you tone health and life … it has been used for 4000 years." Chicory root is the richest source of inulin. It is fascinating, yet not surprising, that many of the food sources of prebiotics have been used for millennia. Today you can find "chicory root" as a functional food ingredient.

Conclusion

Now that you understand prebiotics, the plant based diet, and the prebiotic approach, consider enhancing your diet with some of the natural whole foods we have discussed.

In chapter four, you will learn how prebiotics are used as functional ingredients.

Chapter Four: Prebiotics and Other Fibers as Functional Ingredients

Prebiotics are added to foods to provide a benefit.

Functional Foods

When prebiotics are added to foods they provide a valuable function – the fuel for probiotics in your gut.

Functional foods are foods that have health benefits in addition to their nutritive value. The simplest way to describe a functional food is a food that contains a naturally occurring or added food substance, which when consumed in normal amounts provides beneficial effects which improve health or reduce risk of disease.

Of course there are many natural foods that some argue meet this criteria such as fruits, vegetables, and whole grains which impart health benefits. An example is the tomato which is rich in lycopene that offers a protective benefit. These natural foods require no additional functional ingredients.

An example of a functional food with a functional ingredient is spreads (for bread, potatoes, or other vegetables) containing plant sterols that lower cholesterol, a desirable physiological effect. Another example is foods with omega 3 fatty acids touted to reduce inflammation and reduce triglycerides (blood fats).

The function of prebiotics is to sustain the probiotics thus contributing to digestive and gut health. Once the food is ingested the prebiotics become functional in the gut. This has resulted in a variety of foods designed for digestive health based on the addition of a prebiotic as a functional ingredient. Researchers focusing on gut health and obesity have suggested that by modifying food with prebiotics, it may be possible to impact satiety and gut hormones to assist in weight management.

Glossary

Functional food Foods that have health benefits in addition to their nutritive value.

Synbiotic food Both prebiotic and probiotic ingredients are used in the same food.

Prebiotics in Packaged Foods

Just as you found the market is bulging with products with probiotics, the same is true of foods with prebiotics which have been embraced by the food industry. And they are adding prebiotics to a multitude of foods. For example, you will find prebiotics added to yogurt products (dairy and soy), cottage cheeses, regular cheeses, frozen foods, packaged foods (cereal and energy bars), and baby foods. The labeling lingo for prebiotics is usually very obvious with phases touting their benefits: "prebiotics for digestive health" or "aiding digestion" or simply "prebiotic inulin." For functional foods, the manufacturer should supply the type and amount of prebiotic ingredients per serving.

The Magic of Inulin

Inulin, a natural prebiotic fiber, is found in over 36,000 plants worldwide. It is extracted for use in commercial foods primarily from chicory root, but can also be found in Jerusalem artichokes, agave, and to a lesser extent, dahlia. You may be thinking: "inulin sounds new age to me – what's this all about?" Although inulin is a natural component of many plants, the food industry uses inulin extracted from plants as an ingredient because it is readily available and highly functional. Inulin extract from plants is a food source rather than a manufactured ingredient. Inulin has many functional properties, which not only improve intestinal function, but offer other advantages in foods. Expect to see inulin more often in foods because its magic is to help create foods that are lower in fat calories and yet have a "full fat" mouth feel to the product. It can also help reduce sugar, while providing body, texture, and a neutral tasting fiber. It is a great choice for items such as lower calorie drinkable yogurts. Plus, dairy producers use inulin as a preferred food source for their probiotic cultures. This practice has really caught on in Europe where the trend is to add inulin to a wide variety of foods. As a natural food ingredient, inulin is preferred in making foods with a concentrated dose of a prebiotic.

Pasta, available in so many forms and varieties joins the vast array of foods with prebiotics added as a functional ingredient. Dreamfields Pasta is marketed to help people manage blood glucose levels contains 5 grams of fiber per serving (2 ounces of dry pasta). This is twice the fiber of regular pasta which is around 2 grams for 2 ounces. Included in their fiber blend is the magic ingredient inulin, as well as xanthan gum and pectin, both natural fibers.

www.dreamfieldsfoods.com

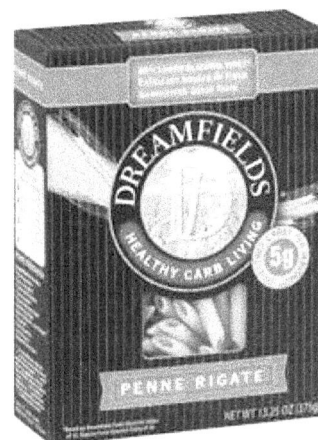

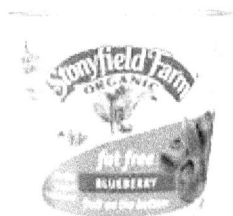

Another example of a food that uses inulin as a functional ingredient is Stonyfield Farm's Fat Free fruit-on-the-bottom yogurts with 2 grams of inulin in each 6 ounce cup. Its function in this food is to promote weight loss and digestive health. Like other dietary fibers, inulin helps suppress hunger, making you feel fuller without adding extra calories. Prebiotic inulin boosts production of the beneficial cultures that naturally reside in your digestive tract and aids digestion.

Kraft and some of its subsidiaries market products designated as *LiveActive* including cottage cheese, cheese sticks, and cheese cubes. All of these products contain 3 grams of prebiotic fiber inulin per serving. The cheese sticks and cubes contain a probiotic *Bifidobacterium lactis.* Very visible on the cartons and packages is the statement "*LiveActive* For Digestive Health."

The intake of inulin from natural food sources has been estimated as 2-8 grams in the US and the estimated intake is higher in Europe. The most common foods contributing inulin are bananas, wheat, onion, garlic, and leek. Our ancestors had a much higher intake of inulin.

How much inulin do you need? It is very individual. Can you get too much? In the scientific literature a dose in excess of 30 grams a day did result in adverse effects. Consuming inulin can result in an increase in your stool mass. The levels vary by individual. Since inulin promotes *bifida* bacteria and may repress the growth of pathogenic bacteria, some people are interested in adding these foods. If you add these foods to your diet, you should do so gradually and assess the results.

Synbiotic Foods

Foods are synbiotic when both prebiotic and probiotic ingredients are used in the same food. Below you will find an example.

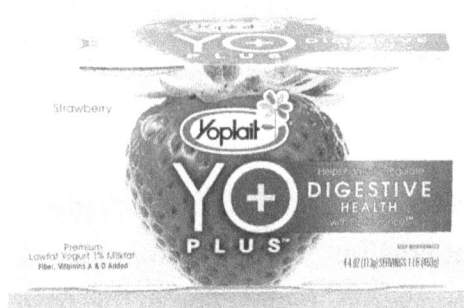

Photo courtesy of Yoplait USA, Inc

YO-PLUS a Yoplait yogurt manufactured by General Mills is an example of a synbiotic food. YO-PLUS™ contains a unique blend of a probiotic and a prebiotic. The blend contains *B. lactis BB-12,* a widely studied probiotic strain, and inulin, a prebiotic. Inulin is the preferred cuisine of *bifidobacteria*. This probiotic/inulin combination helps restore microbial balance in the gut thereby helping to promote overall digestive health.

YO-PLUS also provides S. *thermophilus* and *L. bulgaricus* in the same amounts as in regular Yoplait yogurt. Together all of these ingredients promise to "regulate your digestive health within just one synbiotic food."

Friendship Dairies in New York offers an "all natural lowfat digestive health cottage cheese." It contains *BB 12* (probiotic) with inulin (prebiotic). A 4 ounce serving provides "1 billion live cultures" with 3 grams of inulin. Together they promote "enhanced digestion and bone health."

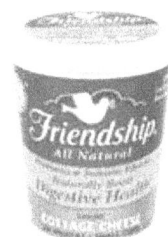

Although the majority of synbiotic foods have been in the dairy category, thanks to the development of creative ways to assure the survival of probiotics such as microencapsulation technology, we now have fruit juices as the carriers. Fruit, especially the "superfruits" such as blueberries, pomegranate, and açai, make an ideal companion for these functional ingredients. Specific fruit compounds as well as their antioxidant profiles contribute to the gut health.

Naked Juice, which touts having "nothing to hide" as they never add sugar or preservatives, launched the first juice with a probiotic in the US in 2007. The probiotic is *Bifidobacterium* (the strain is proprietary information) and the prebiotic is FOS — fructooligosaccharides.

Resistant Starch as a Functional Fiber

Resistant starch is a minor component of starch in some foods (whole grains, potatoes, legumes). As its name implies, it is resistant to digestion until it reaches the colon where it is fermented by resident microorganisms and helps promote human health. Because of its many attributes, food scientists have been making resistant starch from corn, wheat, and potatoes and adding it as a fiber ingredient to foods.

The resistant starch made by starch processing is just like the natural resistant component of starchy foods, it is resistant to normal digestion and it travels on down the GI tract to be fermented in the colon. Numerous rat and human studies have been published with the use of the commercial resistant starches made from high amylase corn which demonstrate that it acts as a fermentable fiber in animals.

Resistant starch is an interesting ingredient that is beginning to be used in a wide array of manufactured foods. You may find this "functional fiber" ingredient in a variety of foods including breads, muffins, cookies, bars, crackers, cereals, and pastas. Why you ask? Well, because you can now enjoy your traditionally low-fiber white bread with the advantages of fiber. The bread still looks the same and has the same familiar taste and texture as regular low-fiber white bread.

In addition to its health benefits from fermentation, the fiber has another favorable effect. When a resistant starch ingredient replaces part of the traditional starch it results in a saving of digestible starch calories. As an insoluble fiber, the labeled caloric contribution is zero calories, but you still get about two calories per gram of the resistant starch when it is fermented in the colon and the resultant fermentation products are utilized by the body for energy. This is still about one-half the calories of standard starch and sugar. You can imagine the potential for reducing calories in some of our favorite foods.

Supplements or Not?

The focus of this book is food rather than supplements. We recommend that if you consider the use of a prebiotic fiber supplement, that you do so only with the guidance of a health professional. Safe consumption levels for prebiotic supplements have not been established. That's why you're safer with a variety of foods and beverages that supply prebiotics naturally. Plus, you get all the other benefits provided by these foods.

Conclusion

Now you know how prebiotics are used as functional ingredients.

Think about your own personal health and individual family members' health status and needs. There may be specific products or foods you want to purchase. And when you get home, will you have room in your fridge and in your cupboards for these wonderful new foods?

In chapter five, we will discuss strategy and we will go into the kitchen.

Chapter Five: Food Safety, the Kitchen, and You

Bacteria — out with the bad; in with the good.

A Clean Kitchen and a Fresh Fridge

The only bacteria you want thriving in your kitchen are the beneficial ones. By keeping a clean kitchen, you guard against pathogenic bacteria so that you avoid food-borne illnesses and protect yourself and your family.

There may be people in your household who are at greater risk for foodborne illness or food poisoning. If they become ill from foodborne bacteria, they are in greater danger of serious health problems and even death. If any of these people eat in your home, you need to be very diligent about checking and discarding spoiled or outdated foods.

At-risk people include:

- pregnant women

- children under 5 years of age

- adults age 65 and older

- people with chronic illnesses (diabetes, kidney disease)

- people with weakened immune systems (patients undergoing cancer treatment, people with organ transplants, and those with HIV infections)

We will teach you how to keep a safe and fresh fridge, including how to interpret date labeling, examine foods for freshness, use storage charts, wash produce. Next, you will learn how to clean your fridge and check the temperature. We also teach you how to keep a healthy pantry with skills for keeping staples safe and pests out. Read on to learn how to sleuth your kitchen for suspect foods. Let's begin with the fridge.

Open the fridge doors and look for "the good, the bad, and the ugly." Your refrigerator is the vault for your fresh food. You will want to keep your fridge heathy and up-to-date. Your schedule depends on your household — if you have someone in your household in one of the at-risk groups, it may require weekly inspection and purging of out of date food or if it's just one or two of you, once a month might suffice. Now let's find "the good, the bad, and the ugly" using your eyes and nose. Let's start by looking at dates on cartons and packages of perishable foods, including dairy, produce, eggs, meat, fish, poultry, and leftovers.

Brittany experienced a shock when she opened her refrigerator door one morning and was bowled over by something that had spoiled and gone super smelly. She tried the quick wipe down method and hoped for the best, but found that the smell would not go away. She checked all of the dairy products for souring and did not find the source. In desperation, she finally emptied and wiped down every shelf and surface. The culprit was black beans in a cardboard take-out carton that had migrated back to a far corner of the refrigerator.

Using Labels and Their Dates

The "sell by" date provided by the manufacturer is meant to guide grocery store staff on when to pull items from the shelf. This means that you are in charge once you get the food home. It is up to you to evaluate how long to keep the food. Check dates on your food items and examine any food beyond its sell by date and discard any food that looks or smells suspicious. Even though the date is passed, the food is likely to be good if you have stored it carefully, especially when you are advised to refrigerate the item. You will see more information on date labels and what they mean in the chart below.

The Scoop on Date Labeling

You will see many versions of date labeling on foods at the grocery store. The labels vary by the kind of food and are used at the discretion of the manufacturer. Note: there is a legal requirement for infant formula and some baby foods.

Sell By	Tells the store how long to display the product for sale. You should buy the product before the date expires.
Use By	The last date recommended for the use of the product while at peak quality. The date has been determined by the manufacturer of the product.
Best If Used By	A "Best if Used By (or Before)" date is recommended for best flavor or quality. It is not a purchase or safety date.
Expires On Do not use after	Legally required for infant formula and some baby foods. Items should be discarded if the date is passed.
Pack Date	Date the item was packed.
Code Date	"Closed or coded dates" are packing numbers for use by the manufacturer.

Examine Foods for Freshness

Dairy Products

Examine your dairy products for changes in texture, smell, and taste. Check foods for growth of molds, fungus, or other unsightly beings. You will see these most commonly on cheeses and cottage cheese. You open the package and realize you kept it way too long – it's green or pink! Yogurt may be safely eaten 7-10 days after the "sell by" date. Milk, usually smells bad if it has "gone bad." The only thing you want to grow in your refrigerator is probiotics! And they are confined in their own cartons.

Ever wonder how long to keep a food. We have compiled storage charts from Food and Drug Administration guidelines and other sources. Find these charts on our website: www.gutinsight.com. Here is a sample chart for the cold case:

Dairy and Non-Dairy — Cold Case Foods

	Fridge	Freezer	Notes
Butter	2-3 weeks	6-9 months	Wrap or cover tightly. Hold only a 2 day supply in the door butter keeper.
Buttermilk	10-14 days		Cover tightly. Separation does not necessarily affect flavor or freshness.
Cheese, cottage	10-15 days		
Cheese, cream	4 weeks		
Cheese, hard (Cheddar, Swiss, Provolone, Gouda)	3-5 months unopened 2 months opened	6 months	
Cheese(Parmesan, Romano)	2-4 months opened	10 months unopened	
Cheese, Ricotta	5 days		
Cream	7-10 days		
Sour cream	2 weeks		
Cream based dips	2 weeks		
Ice cream, ice milk, sherbet		1-2 months	
Milk	1 week or a few days after sell by date		
Kefir	1 week after date, opened 1-2 days		
Yogurt	10-14 days		
Yogurt, frozen		2 months	
Soy and other Non-dairy			
Soy or rice milk	7-10 days		
Tofu	1 week or package date	5 months	
Miso	3 months		

Produce

For produce use your eyes, nose, and touch to evaluate the foods. Apples, fruits and vegetables that have been in your refrigerator for a while that are now turning "soft" or brown should be discarded. Have you ever taken a carrot out of its bag only to have it tilt to the left? It's too old to use. When vegetables are stored too long they change in composition. You will find that old lettuce has gone black on the edges. Greens that are beginning to decompose look like "sludge and slime", and of course these "uglies" should be thrown out.

Most produce is best stored in the refrigerator for enhanced taste and longest shelf life. For most fruit, the best spot is the crisper drawer in a plastic bag and as whole fruit rather than cut up. Exceptions are berries, which should be cleaned and eaten or cleaned and sugared within a day or two of purchase to preserve them. The same applies to ripe summer stone fruit like peaches and nectarines.

For vegetables, refrigeration will extend shelf life. Potatoes, garlic, and onions do better on the cupboard shelf, but you should separate potatoes from the onions and garlic as the gases they naturally produce may accelerate spoilage. Tomatoes are best ripened at room temperature and then consumed. And just for the record, tomatoes are a botanical fruit, but a culinary vegetable, so in this book they are treated as vegetables. See storage charts for fruits and vegetables on our website.

Washing Produce

Before eating or preparing, wash fresh produce under cold running tap water to remove any lingering dirt. This reduces bacteria that may be present. If there is a firm surface, such as on apples or potatoes, the surface can be scrubbed with a brush. Consumers should not wash fruits and vegetables with detergent or soap. These products are not approved or labeled by the Food and Drug Administration for use on foods. You could ingest residues from soap or detergent absorbed on the produce.

When preparing fruits and vegetables, cut away any damaged or bruised areas because bacteria that cause illness can thrive in those places. Immediately refrigerate any fresh-cut items such as salad or fruit for best quality and food safety. Keep fruits separate from raw meat, poultry and seafood while shopping, preparing, or storing. Source: USDA

Eggs

What about eggs and delicatessen products? Well, fresh eggs in the shell may be stored for 4 to 5 weeks, which is not long after their sell by date. Although when you cook eggs, the fresher they are, the better. Store eggs in their original carton in the body of the fridge where it is colder rather than in the door. This will keep them from acquiring odors such as a strong smelling cheese that has been stored nearby. There is some shift in the fluids in the egg during storage and you may not get that "stand up" yolk that you want as the egg ages. To determine if an egg is fresh, place it in a bowl of cold water deep enough to cover it. If the egg is fresh, it will lie on the bottom of the bowl. If the egg stands up and bobs on the bottom, it is less fresh. If the egg floats, according to the USDA: "the egg is old, but it may be perfectly safe to use. Crack the egg into a bowl and examine it for an off-odor or unusual appearance before deciding to use or discard it. A spoiled egg will have an unpleasant odor when you break open the shell, either when raw or cooked."

Meats, Fish, and Poultry

For safety, keep your raw meats, fish, and poultry separated and wrapped so they do not come in contact with other foods or taint the shelves where they are stored. Ground meat should be kept only a day or two before cooking and other fresh meats may be kept three to five days. Fresh fish is best stored for one to two days after purchase by enclosing it in a plastic bag or closed container with a tablespoon of cold water or on ice in a closed container.

Leftovers

How should you store leftovers? The best way is to use containers with lids that fully seal. Foods that come home in the restaurant take-out container will last longer in the fridge if they are transferred to sealed containers. Think about how rice from a Chinese restaurant dries out in the cardboard container. Using sealed containers reduces cross contamination. This will isolate the foods and, if bacteria should start growing, will isolate the bacteria as well. Discard leftovers after storing for two to four days, unless they seem to be spoiling faster. When serving leftovers you should reheat them to 165°F and bring leftover sauces, soups, and gravies to a boil.

Keeping Perishable Food Safe

How does food get "yucky"? Because people taste it and then use the same spoon to taste it again! All those bacteria in the mouth get introduced to a new food source and the bugs "go wild." So please, **Do Not Double Dip**! Your hummus won't even resemble hummus, if you double dip. When you serve the hummus, always remove it from its original container to a serving dish and don't put it back after it's been on the appetizer table.

Not reusing an open container that has contacted mouth fluids is very important when feeding your baby. Remove the baby food from the jar and serve. Put the jar back in the refrigerator for the next time. Discard any food your baby does not eat. It's so much better to be safe than sorry.

Why should you be spending so much time on this? Because you want good bugs in your gut not the ugly ones! And don't you feel better with a clean fridge, one that you are about to fill with whole foods? Most people love having their fridge full of healthy food. It makes them feel empowered. Plus we all like to open a fridge and see numerous choices. This is one reason we go shopping before guests arrive.

Cleaning Your Fridge

Keeping your fridge clean is easier than you might think. Start at the top, removing items, wiping down the shelves with warm (not hot) soapy water. Remove shelves and drawers as needed. A few drops of hand dishwashing soap works best, but a bit of soap with some baking soda will help reduce odors and will not damage the finish on the fridge.

Fridge Cleaning

For a more thorough cleaning, Whirlpool recommends:

"Clean both the refrigerator and freezer compartments about once a month to prevent odors from building up. Wipe up spills immediately. Unplug refrigerator or disconnect power. Remove all removable parts from inside, such as shelves, crispers, etc. Hand wash, rinse, and dry removable parts and interior surfaces thoroughly, using a clean sponge or soft cloth and mild detergent in warm water. Do not use abrasive or harsh cleaners such as window sprays, scouring cleansers, flammable fluids, cleaning waxes, concentrated detergents, bleaches or cleansers containing petroleum products on plastic parts, interior and door liners, or gaskets. Do not use paper towels, scouring pads, or other harsh cleaning tools. These can scratch or damage materials. To help remove odors, you can wash interior walls with a mixture of warm water and baking soda (2 Tbls. to 1 qt (26 g to .95 L) of water). Wash stainless steel and painted metal exteriors with a clean sponge or soft cloth and mild detergent in warm water. Do not use abrasive or harsh cleaners. Dry thoroughly with a soft cloth." www.whirlpool.com

Temperature Matters

Check the temperature of your refrigerator. No thermometer? You can pick one up at the supermarket or hardware store the next time you shop. The safe refrigerator zone is below 40°F. as food spoilage may occur above 40°. (Safe freezer zone is 0°F. and below.) If your power fails, do your best to keep the doors of the refrigerator and freezer closed as much as possible. If the power returns within four hours, the food should be safe if it was cold when the power failed. Recently refrigerated foods that were warm or room temperature will not be safe. When in doubt, discard any food that might have become too warm. For further information on safe food handling during and after a power outage, see the FDA website page: www.cfsan.fda.gov. Search "power outage."

How about storing leftovers? Do they go into the fridge warm or should you let them cool to room temperature before storing? There are lots of myths about this issue. The FDA says: "Refrigerate food quickly because cold temperatures keep most harmful bacteria from multiplying. A lot of people think it will harm their refrigerator to put hot food inside, but it's not true. Hot food won't harm your refrigerator. More important, prompt refrigeration of foods will keep your food and you safer." They continue to say:

- Refrigerate or freeze perishables, prepared food, and leftovers within two hours.
- Divide large amounts of leftovers into shallow containers for quick cooling in the refrigerator.
- Marinate foods in the refrigerator.
- Don't pack the refrigerator too full. Cold air must circulate to keep food safe.

You are safest when you thaw foods in the refrigerator. Alternatively, you may want to thaw a plastic wrapped item outside the refrigerator by immersing it in cold water, changing the water every half hour to keep the temperature cold enough. If you choose to thaw food in the microwave, cook it immediately after it's thawed.

Josh has it easy with his single lifestyle. He is able to dump the take-out containers and check the dates on the dairy foods and go from there. He tries to take care of it before a business trip, since there is nothing worse than coming home from a trip and finding a science experiment and its associated smell in the refrigerator.

Ella tries to keep items in sealed containers, so she checks the dates on dairy products and pays careful attention to what is in her produce drawers.

Kelly has not yet developed the routine of repackaging leftovers in closed containers, so she often finds herself with a serious garbage bag, dumping all the old, smelly food at once. She finds she does this most often just before she puts away foods she has brought home from the supermarket.

The Pantry or Storage Cabinets

Now that your fridge is clean, let's go to your cupboards and pantry. Having well-stocked and properly organized cabinets is like having money in the bank. All of those prebiotic foods, such as grains in the form of flours, pasta, prepared cereals, and whole grains are found there. Having brown rice, wild rice, cornmeal, couscous, and unusual whole grain flours will add interest to your cooking. Beans and dried peas are also stored in cabinets either as whole beans or in cans. While there is a taste advantage to soaking and cooking beans from scratch, you cannot beat the convenience of canned beans. Coffee, tea, and also soy foods in aseptic packaging as well as nuts and unopened nut butters may be safely stored in cabinets.

Pantries have their own shelf life issues. Oh my, for cereals and grains, where do those little bugs come from? They come with the grains from the field. Use the "best before" dates as a guide. Grains and cereals do attract bugs. If you have a small household, it's best not to buy the 42 ounce oatmeal, rather buy the 18 ounce, so you can use it all before the "best before" date. To check your pantry foods for bugs, look for spider-web-like material in the corners of boxes, and small moths larvae moving in the flour or cornmeal. Toss out the infested food. To contain and prevent infestation of other foods, store in a sealed container. Reused glass jars work well as long as the seal on the lid is secure. Traps that attract the bugs and are safe for kitchen use will eventually get rid of the bugs. For expert information, search "Pantry pests UC Davis" in your web browser.

Some items you find in your cupboards may need to go into the refrigerator. You might put dried fruits in the fridge just to keep them out of harm's way. Nuts will keep longer in the fridge by preventing the oils from going rancid. Peanut butter, depending on brand, may be labeled "refrigerate after opening."

Your pantry should be cool, dry, and dark. For the best shelf life, store foods in metal, plastic, or glass containers. Freshness dating applies to canned and dried foods. See storage chart for staples on our website.

Food Preparation

The Clean Kitchen

As you prepare your meals and snacks, we want you to do so in as safe a manner as possible. Earlier in this chaper you learned about when to toss past-date foods. Keep those guidelines in mind as you prepare foods. We recommend frequent hand washing as you handle your food and keeping condiment containers clean.

Cutting Board Controversy: Which is best wood or plastic?

Cutting up foods in preparation for cooking deserves attention. You need to ensure that you are not risking a bout of food-borne illness due to pathogenic bacteria contaminating your cutting boards. The bacteria may be harbored in those boards from a raw food source. Follow these guidelines to ensure safety:

- Use separate boards — one for meat, poultry, and fish, another for fruits and vegetables (although some people like to separate aromatic vegetables like onion from fruits). Separate boards protect against cross contamination.
- Either wood or plastic boards are safe when carefully cleaned and maintained, but some researchers found wood safer.
- Wash boards with hot water and liquid dishwashing detergent and allow to air dry or dry with paper towel. Plastic may be cleaned in the dishwasher.

Bad Bugs on Produce

Here is a summary of tips to make sure that your salad is bug-free and to minimize the possiblity of illness-causing bacteria on your produce.

At the store or produce market	Choose fruits and vegetables without blemishes. Choose produce that is handled the least.
In the kitchen	Store produce that can stand the cold in the refrigerator. (Exceptions are onions, garlic, potatoes, turnips). Wash your hands frequently when you are preparing food. Thoroughly wash fruits and vegetables in lukewarm water before eating. (Commercial produce washes are not recommended). Keep protein foods like meat, fish, poultry and eggs away from produce. Trim any areas on produce that are blemished, bruised, or damaged as well as the stem. Produce that has been washed should be dried with a towel or spun in a salad spinner before returning it to the refrigerator. Try using a salad spinner for more than just lettuce. Greens and leeks will be easier to clean if you spin them. Spinning removes excess moisture and more sand and dirt than other methods.

Microwave Safety

Microwave ovens do not always heat food enough to kill pathogenic bacteria. When heating leftovers, USDA recommends that the food reach 165°F throughout. This can be achieved by cutting the food into pieces and stirring once or twice in the reheating process to avoid any remaining cold spots.

What's Next?

Having a clean refrigerator, pantry, and kitchen with safe foods is a kind of health insurance. Now that you have tossed, cleaned, and sorted, you are ready to restock with probiotic and prebiotic foods.

Chapter Six: Probiotic and Prebiotic Shopping

Go directly to the cold case for probiotics and go to the produce section for prebiotic vegetables.

Probiotic Shopping

Now that your kitchen is in good shape, it is time to shop for food emphasizing those foods that contain probiotics and prebiotics. In this chapter, you will learn to shop for new foods — how to recognize them, learn when they are in season, and learn where to find them in the supermarket. You will also find out about options for shopping like farmers' markets, produce delivery services, and community supported agriculture.

When you are shopping for probiotic laden foods go directly to the refrigerated cases where you will find yogurts with live cultures, kefir with live cultures (dairy and soy). You will also find many other products with live cultures. To keep cultures live and active, all must be refrigerated.

Start with Yogurt

Yogurt is the simplest and most traditional food with probiotics. The process of making yogurt uses *L. bulgaricus* and *S. thermophilous* as starter cultures that change pasteurized milk to yogurt by means of fermentation. The same process is used on soymilk to make soy yogurt. After the fermentation process with starter cultures, additional live active cultures are added – *L. acidophilous, L. casei, L. rhamnosus, B. bifidum.*

If you are trying yogurt for the first time, start with a plain yogurt — dairy or soy. Even if you have only used flavored versions in the past, give the plain version a try. A plain version will give you an appreciation for the original tart taste of the product. Once you are familiar with the tart taste, you may desire to create with your own additions such as honey, fresh or frozen fruit, fruit juice, jam, vanilla, or maple syrup. You may later consider selecting specialty yogurts depending upon your needs for digestive health. Josh, Ella and Kelly illustrate how they select specialty yogurts for their digestive health.

Josh had tried a probiotic supplement designed for irritable bowel and finding relief he was ready to try a specialty yogurt. He liked it, found it effective and now he makes it a habit to eat a carton each day of yogurt designed for digestive health which contains a unique blend of probiotics and inulin a prebiotic. He has found this keeps him regular without the embarrassing episodes he was experiencing.

Ella has a new life since visiting with the nutritionist and finding she can be free of constipation by eating a specialty yogurt daily and making sure she gets plenty of prebiotics. She has experimented with how much of the specialty yogurt she needs and found she was able to gradually reduce from the initial two four-ounce cartons a day to just one carton a day and sometimes just one half carton. She likes mixing it with a plain yogurt.

Kelly is following the advice of her nutritionist with her "health smart" shopping list. Now treated for her excessive gas and bloating she is "happy as a clam" on her new pattern of eating. Allergic to cow's milk protein, she selects her live natural cultures from a variety of soy-based yogurts and smoothies making sure she takes one serving each day.

Beyond Yogurt

There are many other choices for foods with live active cultures of probiotics beyond yogurt. The products are proliferating in the cold case. Bars, juices, specialty cheeses and cottage cheese, smoothies, and child-friendly products.

Here is the short list of foods with live cultures from the cold case, which you will also find in our Full Shopping List on our web site www.gutinsight.com.

Cold Case (Dairy, soy, or other)
Yogurt
Specialty yogurts for digestive health
Yogurt smoothies
Kefir
Cottage cheese and other cheeses with probiotics
Probiotic juice
Probiotic bars

A Word about Miso

Miso is a paste used in Asian cooking that is made by fermenting soybeans and grains with molds, yeast, and bacteria. We often see miso included in lists of probiotic foods in popular articles, but we have not found enough scientific evidence to officially include it in our list of probiotic food sources. The bacteria and yeasts used in miso need further study.

Miso is known as a health food and it can be a savoury addition to your existing recipes. If there are live bacteria, heating the miso would destroy them — so add it to a food that is already cooked. It is quite salty and comes in several varieties. The classic recipe is miso soup from Japanese cuisine, but we also suggest that you use it to top grilled fish or add it to cooked polenta or other grains that have not yet been salted.

Prebiotic Shopping

Two important prebiotic staples are onions and garlic. They are available year round, versatile in their uses, easy to store, and have additional health benefits. Keep them on hand in your kitchen. Include other onion-family members (shallots, green onions, and leeks) when they are available.

Prebiotic Produce in Season

We have listed **prebiotic stars** in the chart below. The chart uses an asterisk (*) to indicate the best months to shop for these foods. Other foods have been mentioned in scientific literature, but have not been studied thoroughly enough to assure their prebiotic effects. These seasonality of these **prebiotic potentials** are designated with bullets (•).

Buying produce in-season means that you are getting the plant when it is at its full potential. In-season foods are often grown locally and have not traveled long distances. However, our supermarkets today have such a wide variety of produce imported from all over the world and you might not know what is in season. A local farmer's market is of course the answer, for they do not import. They grow it themselves! For information on seasonality in your specific geographical area in the US, see: Field to Plate: What's In Season in Your Region? www.fieldtoplate.com/guide.php

And if you can't buy in season, but really want that food, then check out the canned and frozen sections as an alternative.

And if you can't buy in season, but really want that food, then check out the canned and frozen sections as an alternative.

Vegetables	J	F	M	A	M	J	J	A	S	O	N	D	All Year
Artichoke			*	*	*	*				*			
Asparagus			*	*	*								
Burdock													*
Chicory root													*
Dahlia tubers									*	*	*		
Dandelion greens			*	*	*								
Endive (chicory, wiltoof, endive)													•
Garlic													*
Greens (spinach, chard, collard, sorrel, mustard, beet, turnip, leafy greens, etc.)							•	•	•	•	•	•	
Jerusalem artichoke	*	*	*							*	*		
Jicama	•	•	•	•	•					•	•	•	
Leeks									*	*	*	*	
Dandelion greens													*
Onions													*
Onions, sweet													*
Onions, green													*
Salsify or oyster plant	*	*								*	*		
Shallots													*
Tomatoes							•	•	•				

Fruits	J	F	M	A	M	J	J	A	S	O	N	D	All Year
Apples	•	•	•	•					•	•	•		
Bananas													*
Berries				•	•	•	•	•					
Raisins													•

As research continues, more foods may be identified as having a prebiotic effect. In the meantime, continue to purchase a variety of plant-based foods. They have nondigestible carbohydrates that may prove to be prebiotic and they have other health benefits.

Whole Grains

Whole wheat, barley, and rye are prebiotic stars. Whole wheat is the most common prebiotic food in the American diet. You will find whole wheat in bread, pasta, crackers, tortillas, couscous, cracked wheat or bulgur, wheat berries, and whole wheat flour. Look for barley in a bag, often near the beans and peas on the lower shelves. On the bread and cracker aisles find whole grain options for rye and barley.

Whole Grain Prebiotic Stars

Whole wheat

Barley

Rye

Other Foods – Prebiotic Potentials

For **prebiotic potentials**, choose other grains like oats, brown rice, polenta, corn meal, or popcorn. Look in the frozen food section where you can always find corn and may find brown rice in individual packets ready to microwave or heat on the stovetop.

Prebiotic Potentials

Oats

Brown rice

Whole grain corn

Buckwheat

Beans, lentils, peas

Honey

Flaxseed

Almonds

Beans, Lentils, and Peas

Beans are a rich source of protein. Although there has been sparse investigation on the prebiotic effect of their carbohydrates, some scientists list beans and lentils as prebiotics. We consider them prebiotic potentials. A great variety is available. Try black, pinto, white, kidney, garbanzo, lima, and black-eyed peas. You can find them in cans, bulk bins, or in packages. Lentils and split peas may be found in bulk bins or packages. The soup section has bean soups, such as minestrone, lentil, and split pea. The deli section will also have bean salads.

Legumes or Pulses

Plants in the botanical family Fabaceae (formerly Leguminosae) are those dried edible beans, lentils and peas that are excellent sources of fiber and have prebiotic potential.

Beans include adzuki, Anasazi, appaloosa, atebo, black or turtle, calypso, canary, cannellini or white kidney, cranberry, Dutch brown, European soldier, fava, flageolet, great northern, Jacob's cattle, kidney, lima or butter, mung, navy, pink, pinto, small red, trout, white marrow.

Soybeans include whole, edamame, and roasted soy nuts.

Chickpeas include kabuli (found in bulk and canned in US). They may be called garbanzo, ceci, cici, cheechee, Bengal gram, gram, chana, pois chicke, shihu, chola, pois chiche, gran, kabuli, channa, or safaid beans.

Desi (small, darker seeds and a rough coat) may be called kala chana, Bengal gram, gram, chana, pis chiche, or chihu. When split they resemble yellow split peas and may be called split desi chickpea, Bengal gram, yellow gram, gram, chana pois, or chicke shihu.

Lentil varieties include brown, black or beluga, French green, red, yellow split, white.

Peas include green and yellow split, lupini beans, black-eyed pea, pigeon pea.

Note: **Jicama**, the root of the yam bean plant, is in the legume family and contains inulin.

Honey, Flaxseed, and Almonds

Honey, flaxseed, and almonds are **prebiotic potentials**. They are most often found in the baking section, but could be located in the produce section.

Super Foods

What are super foods? Is there a list of super foods?

Well, yes, sort of, there are foods that have enough science behind them that some feel they qualify as super foods. The truth of the matter is that some foods are studied more than others. Scientists study specific foods when there is funding to do so and those foods have much more research data than others. Often advisory and marketing boards for a particular food have a lot of money to spend on research. This contributes to the total body of science on foods, nutrition, and health.

We think any food that is a whole plant food is a super food. Why? Because plant foods are chock-full of potent antioxidants, fibers, phytochemicals, phenols, and other natural ingredients that protect you and promote your health.

A plant has to protect itself from different enemies and environmental conditions. Scientists have found that some of their protective chemicals also protect you. Plus many of the protective nutrients actually are responsible for their color. Perhaps you have always been told to eat the deep yellow and deep green vegetables. The reason is that carotenoids (carotene) color the vegetable — consider the carrot. Another carotene is lycopene which gives the tomato its red color.

Super foods come from the ground or are picked from a tree or vine!

Josh, Ella, and Kelly Go Shopping

Josh

Josh, the successful young businessman, keeps his shopping list on his Blackberry with a weekly reminder to go to the store. In addition to the specialty yogurt he has for breakfast, he also enjoys plain yogurt topped with granola as a nighttime snack. He knows from his nutrition counseling that prebiotics are important too, so he always has bananas on the list. Then he buys whatever else is in season. Josh is progressing to a healthier diet and with small steps. He still relies on "take-out "for most of his meals.

Josh's short list:

    Specialty yogurt

    Kefir

    Granola with whole grains

    Almonds

    Bananas, apples, berries

    Espresso coffee

    Take out from the deli

Ella

Ella, the active woman in her fifties, is trying to follow her nutritionist's advice. She eats specialty and plain yogurt daily and has several good helpings of prebiotic rich foods and plenty of fluids as well.

Ella's shopping list is in her purse and she adds to it as she thinks of things she needs. She always has a basic grocery list. She goes into the produce section with an open mind and buys whatever looks the best. She is a creative cook and often makes her meals from scratch. She prepares fish, poultry, or meat along with two vegetables and whole grain side dishes for an evening meal. For a lighter meal she enjoys a salad with whatever fresh ingredients she has on hand topped with parsley and canned beans.

Ella's basic list:

> Specialty yogurt
>
> Yogurt plain
>
> Fresh fruits
>
> Fresh vegetables
>
> Onions, shallots, garlic
>
> Whole grains
>
> Canned beans
>
> Canned tomatoes
>
> Fresh fish, poultry or meat
>
> Green and black tea

Kelly

Kelly, a college student who is trying to lose weight, does her best to follow the advice of her nutritionist with her "lifestyle" shopping list.

Allergic to cow's milk protein, she selects her live natural cultures from a variety of soy based yogurts and smoothies making sure she has one serving each day. She is eating more fruits and vegetables, often relying on canned or frozen versions as she just doesn't get to the store as often as she would like and uses her microwave oven most of the time. Her list supports her lifestyle as a student with quick and easy foods. When she shops, she is focused and in control and does not deviate to the aisles with the tempting salty or sweet snacks. She knows these snacks are "very occasional foods." She is thinking about some simple cooking, but is waiting for the right time to begin.

Kelly's "lifestyle" list

- Soy yogurt
- Soy smoothies
- Fresh eggs
- Packaged meats
- Whole grain pocket bread
- Hummus
- Lettuce
- Onion
- Fresh or canned fruits (in light syrup)
- Fresh, frozen or canned vegetables
- Canned tuna and salmon
- Tofu burgers

Conclusion

Probiotic shopping is easy and straightforward. Just select foods with live active cultures. Prebiotic shopping is more challenging since these foods are found in various sections of the market. You are now knowledgeable about these food sources, so the skill of shopping will naturally follow. You'll need to shop for other foods, so in the next chapter we visit markets, provide shopping lists, and give you tips to hone your shopping skills.

Chapter Seven: Mindful Marketing

Hunting and gathering are instincts as old as mankind and modern shoppers share characteristics with their ancestors: they track and pounce.

The modern hunter-gatherer shops at supermarkets, super stores, small neighborhood stores, farmers markets, and online. Some shoppers order boxes filled with organic produce and dairy products which appear each week on their front steps.

There are all kinds of shoppers, some meander through the market getting a feel for the territory and its offerings, others are shopping with their smart phone in hand swooping in and scooping up items while traveling their familiar path. You may be somewhere in the middle, going to the market with half an idea of what you need and shopping with the purpose of getting out of there as soon as possible. In this chapter we focus on mindful marketing, shopping with ease and purpose, while making it as enjoyable as possible. In fact we will introduce you to some new, exciting ways to shop.

The golden rule for mindful marketing is to stay focused on the task. Begin with a list. The goal is to shop for natural whole foods, and not just those found in the produce section, but those on the shelves as well. Try visiting the produce section first, then the aisles known as the "inner zone" of the store where you find the canned and packaged foods. Later, shop the cold case for dairy or soy items, and finally the perishables — fish, poultry, and meat. Lists of foods for each section make mindful marketing easy and help you stay focused.

As you map out your foray into the store emphasizing the natural whole foods and ignoring the highly processed foods, you'll need the healthiest route. Let's face it, there are many of distractions.

The Center Aisles

Often canned fruits, vegetables, and beans are a convenient alternative to the fresh version and with very little change in their nutritive value. Canning processes preserve nutrients and provide a longer shelf life. Canned items for making quick meals might include beans, tomatoes and tomato sauces, red peppers, beets, olives, artichoke hearts, hearts of palm, water chestnuts, bamboo shoots, chilis, pineapple, mandarin oranges, and other selected canned fruit. In the soup section, shop for stocks such as chicken, beef, or vegetable to build soups with fresh foods, beans, and grains.

Go to the bread aisle. Look for breads with part or all whole grains listed as one of the first ingredients. Be aware of additives. In some European countries, there are purity laws for bread that limit the ingredients to grain, water, yeast and salt. That is a good place to start with bread and if you find too many additives, choose a simpler version. Breads come in all kinds of whole grain options, so consider rye, barley, wheat, oat, and more exotic grains always choosing primarily whole grains.

You may also find staples like pasta, rice, and other whole grains in the center aisles as well as dried beans and peas.

Grains	Beans and Peas (canned or dried)
Bread, whole grain (rye, barley, wheat, oat, buckwheat)	Beans (black, pinto, garbanzo, kidney, lima, soy, small red, small white, cannellini, Black eyed peas, exotics)
Pasta, whole grain	
Bulgur, wheat berries	
Polenta, cornmeal	Lentils (red, brown, French, beluga black)
Tortillas	
Flours, whole grain (pastry)	Split peas (yellow, green)
Rice, brown	
Oats	Edamame (soy beans, cold case or frozen)
Wild rice	
Exotic grains (spelt, quinoa)	
Cereals, prepared whole grain	
Barley, pearled	

On the baking aisle, you will find whole grain flours and cornmeal as well as nuts and chocolate. Nuts and seeds are good sources of protein, fiber and beneficial fats, so look for peanuts, almonds, cashews, pistachios, walnuts, pecans, hazelnuts, macadamias, sunflower seeds, pine nuts, sesame seeds, pumpkin seeds, and nut butters made from those nuts. (Peanuts actually are legumes, but we consider them a "culinary nut" — just as the tomato, a fruit, is a culinary vegetable). Some of these seeds will also be available as ingredients in breads. Baking supplies are important not only if you bake, but also for other cooking. Cornstarch and tapioca might be added to savory dishes and you will find many whole grain baking mixes for muffins and pancakes. Chocolate options include cocoa, dark chocolate, and unsweetened chocolate.

Nuts and seeds	Baking and seasoning
Almonds	Flour, whole grain
Cashews	Jam or jelly
Coconuts, fresh	Syrup
Flaxseed	Honey
Hazelnuts	Raisins
Macadamias	Sugar
Peanuts	Baking soda / powder
Pecans	Tapioca
Pine nuts	Vanilla
Pistachios	Yeast
Poppy seeds	Chocolate
Pumpkin seeds	Corn Starch
Sesame seeds	Baking mixes
Sunflower seeds	Carob
Walnuts	
Tahini (ground sesame seeds)	
Nut butters from the above	

Choose condiments to add interest to fresh foods. Consider soy sauce or tamari, vinegars of every sort, olives, olive oil, canola oil, mustard, chutney, salsas, fruit spreads, wasabi, Tabasco or other chili sauce. Skip the aisles that feature less healthy foods like soda, cookies, candy, and heavily processed foods.

Condiments
Vinegar (apple cider, balsamic, red wine, rice, malt)
Mustard
Mayonnaise
Catsup
Worcestershire
Soy sauce / Tamari
Chutney
Salsa
Chili oil or sauce
Wasabi
Horseradish

The Dairy Case

You will find many probiotic foods with "live active cultures" (yogurt, yogurt smoothies, acidophilus milk, kefir, and some cheeses) in the dairy case. Other dairy foods may be on your list as well: milk, cottage cheese, cheese. Dairy alternatives found in this section include soy yogurt with live active cultures, soy yogurt smoothies, soy, rice or nut milk, tofu, tempeh, and miso. Other dairy case foods for your list are eggs, vegetable oil margarine (without trans-fatty acids or hydrogenated oils), dips made of whole foods like hummus, guacamole, and fresh salsas made with vegetables as well as fruits, kim chee (a Korean fermented cabbage salad), and edible seaweeds.

Cold Case (Dairy, soy, or other)
Yogurt
Yogurt smoothies
Kefir
Cottage cheese (check label for live active cultures or prebiotic inulin)
Milk
Acidophilus milk
Cheese
Eggs
Dips
Spreads
Tofu
Miso (soy paste)
Pesto
Salsa

The Freezer

The freezer section is a treasure trove of foods that might be out of season, but were picked at their peak. Look for peas, corn, edamame, black-eyed peas, lima beans, whole grain waffles. Try some frozen berries for building smoothies and fruit crisps.

Freezer
Vegetables
Fruits
Waffles
Whole grains (brown rice)

The Deli

Items in the prepared foods or deli section can be a source of prebiotic ingredients. You might choose bean salads, whole grains salads, vegetables, sandwiches on whole grain breads, and other items that you might not want to make at home. Of course this would be the more expensive choice since deli take-out is as expensive as many restaurants.

Keeping it Fresh

There are methods you can use while shopping to protect the freshness of the foods you are purchasing as well as enhancing food safety to protect the health of those in your household.

Use date labels to choose foods. The Date Labeling chart is available in chapter five and is also available on the website www.gutinsight.com.

Shop the produce section and center aisles first. Leave the dairy case, freezer, and butcher area for last since items from these areas are more perishable. Consider tossing a cold bag into the car with your cloth shopping bags and your list. Then, when you load the groceries into the car, you can shift perishables like meat, dairy products, and eggs into the cold bag. Consider using cold bags for farmers' market items and then head for the conventional grocery store nearby. The produce stays cool and fresh in the car and you have saved a trip.

When you arrive home, be sure to put away those dairy case and freezer items quickly. You should transfer grains to glass containers with sealable lids.

Shopping Alternatives

Farmers' Markets

When you are searching for fresh local food you cannot beat a farmers' market. For a directory of farmers markets, see: www.ams.usda.gov and search "farmers markets." The USDA reports on their website that there are "more than 4,300 farmers markets operating throughout the nation." Not all farmers' markets are included in this directory, so check with local sources for where to find them in your area.

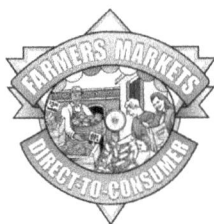

Alternatively, search www.localharvest.org/farmers-markets/ by name or zip code. You can find fresh produce that is locally grown, usually sold at reasonable prices, often organic, and with increased choices. An added bonus is that you might have the chance to meet the grower or get hints from the vendor on preparation.

Home Delivery

Some areas of the US have home delivery of produce. Search your web browser with the terms *produce delivery* and *your city or region name* to find one near you.

Google   produce delivery   Search   Advanced Search
                                               Preferences

Community Supported Agriculture

Some sustainable farms operate with a seasonal subscription. You pay a fee at the beginning of the season for a share of whatever the farmer is able to produce that growing season. This phenomenon is called Community Supported Agriculture (CSA). These vendors supply produce they have grown that is in-season. Subscribers might find surprise items in their box providing the opportunity to try foods that are new to them. Some farms have customers pick up their supply; others deliver to a central location. See: www.localharvest.org/csa.

What's Next?

Shopping mindfully for probiotic and prebiotic foods gets your ready for the next two chapters on food prepararion.

Chapter Eight: Probiotics Quick and Easy

It is your kitchen, not your medicine cabinet, that supports your health.

Try thinking of your kitchen as a place full of possibilities, pleasures, and promise. You should aspire to making your kitchen the place in your home where you can nourish your body with food that is delicious, nutritious, and safe. Whether your cooking skill is that of a novice or of an inspiring chef like Julia Child, this is a worthy and achievable goal.

The foods containing probiotics that we will use here are those that are readily available and minimally processed. They are primarily dairy products and dairy alternatives like soy. Right from the dairy case and with no preparation, you might enjoy yogurt, kefir, soy yogurt, or probiotic soy milk. Talk about "fast food." You can eat these right out of the fridge and they are mostly in a single serving size. Keep in mind that recipes that are cool or at room temperature at serving time keep the beneficial bacteria alive. Cooking kills the probiotic bacteria.

Three Simple Steps

Step 1 The easiest way to introduce foods with probiotics and prebiotics into your life is to begin with breakfast since so many of these foods are compatible with the first meal of the day. Start with a serving of the yogurt of your choice — dairy or soy; plain or flavored. Add a cereal — cooked oatmeal, granola, or a packaged whole grain cereal. Another choice is a whole grain muffin or toast. Add some fresh fruit and you are on your way. Or try the "on the go burrito" with a whole grain tortilla, peanut or other nut butter, and fresh in season fruit.

Step 2 Prepare some easy yogurt based salad dressings to keep on hand and use with fresh produce or a savory sauce to top a side dish. Homemade Ranch Dressing with yogurt is a heathy alternative to bottled store dressing. Ranch can be used as a green salad dressing, a fresh vegetable dip, or a dressing for pasta salad. Honey Yogurt Dressing encourages the addition of fruit to any meal. Make a savory sauce by adding a teaspoon or two of curry powder, chili powder, cumin or other savory spice to each cup of yogurt. Adjust the amount to your taste. Use as a side sauce or garnish for beans, lentils, or vegetable dishes.

Step 3 Indulge in snacks such as fruit smoothies made with yogurt or kefir, fruit cups using sweetened berries and yogurt, parfaits with yogurt, fruit or fruit puree, granola and nuts. Try one of these as a four o'clock pick-me-up snack. You will get protein, calcium, vitamins, and fiber as well as the lift you need to maintain your energy level.

How Our Friends Use Probiotics at Breakfast

Let's see how our friends Josh, Ella, Kelly and Brittany integrate these and other healthy foods into their busy lifestyles.

Take-Out King

Since Josh is the quintessential take-out king, his probiotic food of choice is a specialty yogurt. For breakfast, he keeps some muffins from a local bakery in the freezer that he can thaw for a few seconds in the microwave and have with his carton of yogurt.

Intrepid Eater

Ella chooses a specialty yogurt and has a breakfast that is similar to Josh's since she lives alone. Sometimes she whips up a smoothie in her blender using fresh or frozen berries and bananas or makes whole grain pancakes from scratch.

Novice Cook

Kelly, the novice cook and college student, sticks to boxed cereal and a carton of soy yogurt each morning. This keeps her hunger at bay and provides good nutrition until lunch.

Health Nut

Brittany, the health nut, is a health conscious eater and exerciser. Her probiotic food choice is plain lowfat yogurt, which she has for breakfast with granola.

Breakfast Recipes

Here are a few recipes to help you with Step 1.

Yogurt and Granola Breakfast

    8 ounces plain yogurt (dairy or soy)
    1 T ground flaxseed
    ½ C granola of choice
    Fresh fruit (optional)

Mix together in a bowl. Eat and enjoy.

Yogurt and Oatmeal Breakfast

    ¾ C cooked oatmeal (follow package directions for 1 serving)
    ¼ C plain yogurt (dairy or soy)
    ¼ C fresh fruit such as berries, peaches, or other fruit
    1 T nuts of choice (optional)
    Honey drizzled on top (optional to taste)

Mix together and enjoy.
Note: Canned, frozen, or stewed dried fruit may also be used.

Breakfast Burrito to Go

    1 whole grain tortilla
    2 T peanut butter or other nut butter
    1/3 C fresh fruit (banana, kiwi, berries, peaches, nectarines)

Spread the peanut butter on the tortilla. Add the fruit. Roll and go.

Salad Dressing Recipes

These recipes for Step 2 may also be used as dipping sauces for vegetables or fruits.

Ranch Dressing

    1 C mayonnaise of choice
    1 C plain yogurt (dairy or soy)
    1-2 small cloves garlic or 1 t garlic powder
    1 t dried onion powder
    1/2 t salt
    2 t dried parsley

Combine all ingredients and store in glass jar in refrigerator.

Honey Yogurt Fruit Salad Dressing

    1/2 c. plain yogurt (dairy or soy)
    2 T honey
    Crushed or minced mint leaves to taste

Mix well. Top a fruit salad. Use as a dip for fresh fruit.

Option: Poppy seeds may be added for color and texture.

Snack Recipes

All ages will enjoy these recipes for Step 3.

Fruit Smoothie

    1 C frozen berries of any sort
    1 banana
    1 C fruit - peaches, apricots, berries, , cherries, applesauce (fresh in-season preferred)
    1 C yogurt (dairy or soy)(plain for a tart smoothie, flavored for sweeter)
    1/4 to 1/2 C fruit juice of choice, milk, or soymilk (enough to keep the blender going)

Add ingredients to blender in order.

Variation: use frozen banana (that has been peeled, cut into large chunks and frozen in a plastic bag) in place of the frozen berries and use fresh berries or other fruit. Frozen fruit is preferable to adding ice.

Yogurt Parfaits

3 cups vanilla yogurt (dairy or soy)

2 cups ripe nectarines or peaches

1 cup fresh berries

2 cups granola of choice or mix of granola and chopped nuts

6 parfait glasses (or wine goblets or drinking glasses)

Combine cut strawberries with blueberries. Spoon 1/4 cup yogurt into a glass, then a layer of berries, then 2 tablespoons of granola, then another layer of yogurt and another of berries. Top with 1 tablespoon of granola. Serve immediately or refrigerate up to 6 hours.

Berry Yogurt Cups

1-1/2 C fresh strawberries, cleaned and sliced

1-1/2 C fresh blueberries

1 carton (8 oz.) vanilla yogurt or plain yogurt with added vanilla

Honey, maple syrup or sugar to taste and depending on the yogurt used

1/4 t ground cinnamon

Divide fruit among four individual serving dishes. Combine the yogurt, sweetener of choice and cinnamon in a bowl; spoon over fruit.

For more recipe sources, see our website www.gutinsight.com.

Making Your Own

Yogurt Cheese

Line a large strainer or colander with cheesecloth. Place this over a bowl and then pour in the yogurt. Do not use yogurt made with the addition of gelatin. Gelatin will inhibit whey separation. Let it drain overnight covered with plastic wrap. Empty the whey from the bowl. Fill a strong plastic storage bag with some water, seal and place over the cheese to weigh it down. Let the cheese stand another 8 hours after which it is ready to use. The flavor is similar to a sour cream with a texture of a soft cream cheese. A pint of yogurt will yield approximately 1/4 lb. of cheese. The yogurt cheese has a shelf life of approximately 7-14 days when wrapped and placed in the refrigerator and kept at less than 40°F.

Use yogurt cheese to top a baked potato or a side dish. It can also be used as a base for dips.

Homemade Dairy Yogurt

For those of you who are interested, here is information on making yogurt at home.

www.ianrpubs.unl.edu/epublic/pages/publicationD.jsp?publicationId=525

www.extension.missouri.edu/explore/hesguide/foodnut/gh1183.htm

www.uga.edu/nchfp/publications/nchfp/factsheets/yogurt.html

Yogurt Makers

Search "yogurt makers" in your favorite web search engine.

Starter Cultures

Many home cooks use commercial yogurt to start their homemade yogurt. Starter cultures are also available from internet sources. Search "yogurt starter cultures" or see www.danlac.com.

Homemade Kefir

Here is an authoritative source on making your own kefir.

www.uga.edu/nchfp/publications/nchfp/factsheets/kefir.html

What's Next?

Now that you have ideas about using probiotic foods in your meals, let's move on to using plant-based prebiotic foods.

Chapter Nine: Prebiotics, the Familiar and the Exotic

You don't have to cook fancy or complicated masterpieces — just good food from fresh ingredients. Julia Child

Think about a food that gives you pleasure. It could be summer tree fruits like apricots, cherries, and nectarines. It could be fall fruits like apples and pears, or fall vegetables like butternut squash or sweet potatoes. Or spring melons. Surely you have a favorite that you not only enjoy eating, but also looking at it. Picture a bowl of your favorite – it is as aesthetic as a vase of flowers.

In this chapter, we will discuss the use of the familiar and introduce you to exotic prebiotic foods. We include prebiotic stars and potentials. We will teach you about them with a guide that includes photographs, descriptions, and information on how to select, store and use them. We have included all the pertinent information we can find on these foods. Simple recipes are provided to encourage their use. Plus we provide internet sites that have the kind of recipes you might consider using if you are feeling adventurous. We also have these and other recipes on our web site (www.gutinsight.com).

Familiar Prebiotic Foods

Familiar prebiotic foods are those that should be available in any well-stocked supermarket when in season. Prebiotics stars are designated with an asterisk, prebiotic potentials are without one.

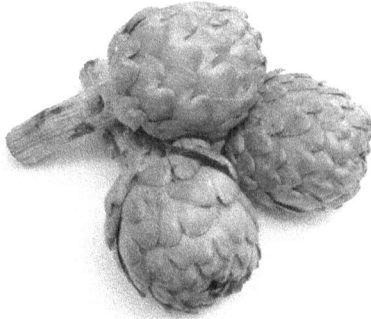

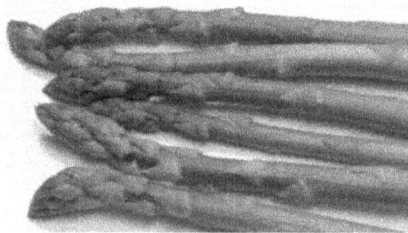

Artichoke*	Season: March-June, October
	Family: *Asteraceae*
	Genus and Species: *Cynara scolymus*
	Native to Mediterranean. Grown in North America.
	Eaten by themselves, used in soups and salads, or stuffed, there are many simple and extravagant preparations for artichokes. They are also available canned for out-of-season use.
	Find out everything about artichokes with recipes at www.artichokes.org
Also known as the globe artichoke.	Find further recipes at www.oceanmist.com.
	Learn how to eat an artichoke with an online video at www.oceanmist.com

Asparagus*	Season: March-June
	Family: *Asparagaceae*
	Genus and Species: *Asparagus officinalis*
	Native to Europe, Middle East, and Africa. Grown in North America.
	Rinse asparagus, break off stem ends or cut off small edge if trimmed. If skin on stems is thickened, use a vegetable peeler to remove part of it. Arrange in one layer in an ovenproof pan, drizzle olive oil, add salt and pepper to taste and roast at 350 degrees for 10-20 minutes depending on size. For recipes and "asparagus tips" see www.calasparagus.com.

Jerusalem artichoke*	Season: November-March
	Family: *Asteraceae*
	Genus and Species: *Helianthus tuberosus L.*
	Native to eastern North America.
	Jerusalem artichokes may be eaten cooked or raw, peeled or unpeeled (although if they are used unpeeled, they should be thoroughly scrubbed). They are often prepared just like potatoes.
Also known as sunchoke, sunroot, topinambour.	When served raw, they should be peeled and sliced into sticks and placed in ice water to crisp. They may then be lightly salted and used like radishes or water chestnuts. For further recipes see www.samcooks.com.

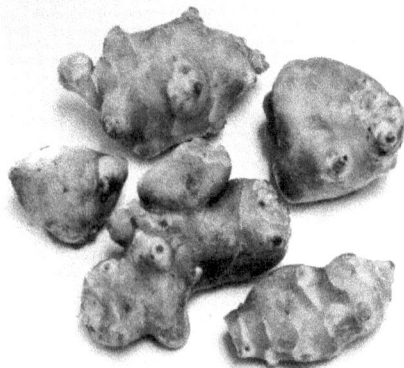

Jicama

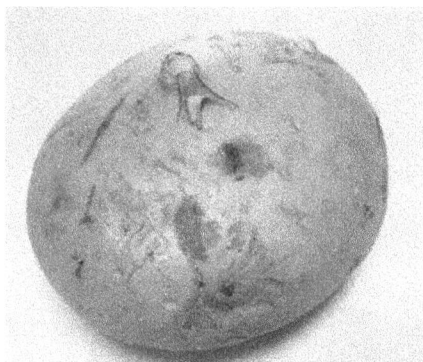

Also known as yam bean root, Mexican potato, Mexican turnip.

Season: November-May

Family: *Fabaceae*

Genus and Species: *Pachyrhizus erosus*

Native to Mexico and Central America.

May be used raw or cooked. Peel root and cut into dice or sticks for appetizers or in salads combined with fruits or vegetables.

When cooked can be a substitute for water chestnuts.

See all about jicama
www.extension.iastate.edu/healthnutrition
/foodrecipeactivity/food/jicama.htm

Onion*

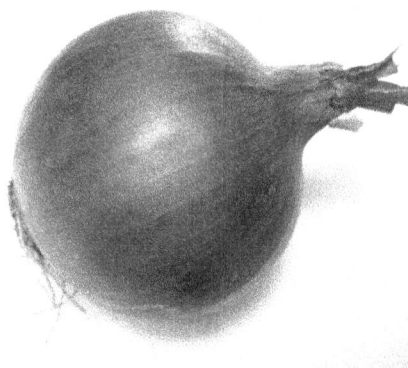

Season: Year round

Family: *Alliaceae*

Genus and Species: *Allium cepa* and many other species.

Native to China, Iran, Europe, and North America.

Onions may be used in nearly any savory dish.

Leek*

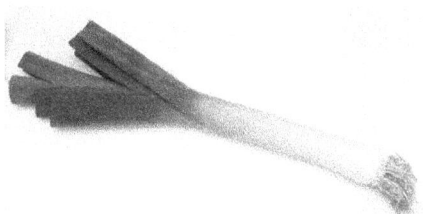

Season: September through April at peak but available year round.

Family: *Alliaceae*

Genus and Species: *Allium ampeloprasum var. porrum*

Native to: Western Asia, Mediterranean.

Trim root end of each leek. Slice lengthwise. If there is excess sand, rinse once now. Slice into half inch half-rounds from the bottom. As you reach darker green outside leaves, discard the course dark parts and continue to slice and keep using the white and light green inside parts. Rinse the half-rounds in a colander or salad spinner.

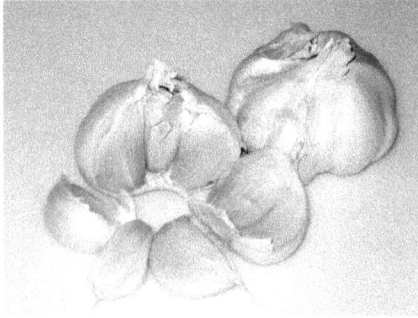

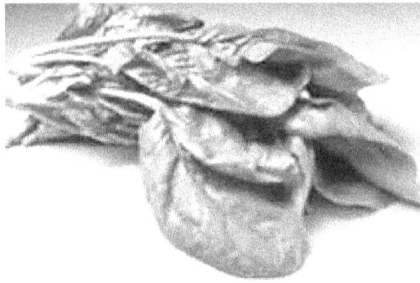

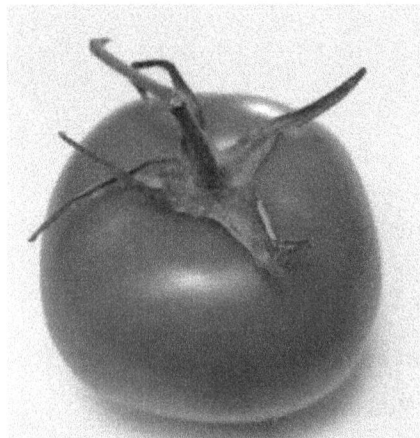

Garlic*	Season: Year round
	Family: *Alliaceae*
	Genus and Species: *Allium sativum* and many other species.
	Find bulb garlic or consider jarred garlic puree or dried garlic. Store fresh garlic at room temperature in a dark place with some ventilation. Store separately from potatoes.

Spinach	Season: Year round
	Family: *Amaranthaceae*
	Genus and Species: *Spinacia oleracea*
	Prepare spinach by rinsing and running through a salad spinner to ensure that all the sand is removed.

Tomato	Season: Year round
	Family: *Solanaceae*
	Genus and Species: *Solanum lycopersicum L.* or *Lycopersicon lycopersicum, Lycopersicon esculentum*
	Native to Central, South, and southern North America from Mexico to Peru.
	Store tomatoes at room temperature. Many varieties are available.

Banana*

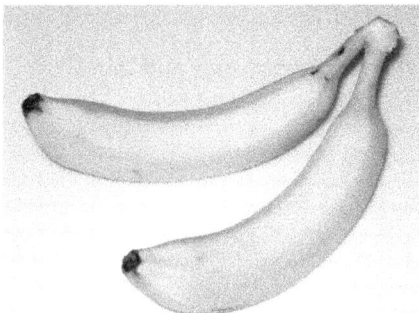

Season: Year round

Family: *Musaceae*

Genus and Species: *Musa acuminata* or the hybrid *Musa × paradisiaca*, a cultigen)

Native to the tropical region of Southeast Asia and Australia. Cultivated throughout the tropics.

Apple

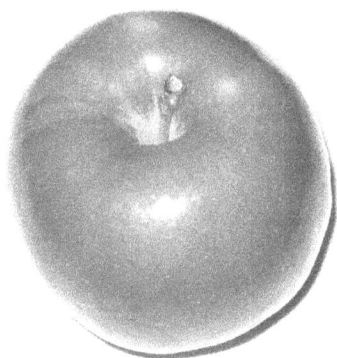

Season: Year round, best in fall

Family: *Rosaceae*

Genus and Species: *Malus domestica*

Native to Central Asia, grown all over the world.

See www.usapple.org.

Berries

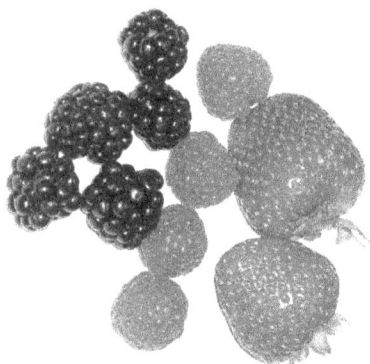

Season: Spring

Family: *Rosaceae*

Genus and Species:

> Black raspberries *Rubus occidentalis*
>
> Blackberry: *Rubus ursinus, Rubus argutus, Rubus fruticosus*
>
> Boysenberry: *Rubus ursinus x idaeus*
>
> Raspberry: *Rubus strigosus*
>
> Strawberry: *Fragaria × ananassa*

See www.oregon-berries.com.

North American Raspberry & Blackberry Association www.raspberryblackberry.com.

Blueberries	Season: Summer
	Family: *Ericaceae*
	Genus and Species: *Vaccinium corymbosum* and many other species
	Native to North America.
	See www.blueberrycouncil.com.

Cranberries	Season: Fall and winter
	Family: *Ericaceae*
	Genus and Species: *Vaccinium macrocarponcetin*
	Native to North America.
	See www.library.wisc.edu/guides/agnic/cranberry/cranuse.htm.

Raisins	Season: year round
	Family: *Vitaceae*
	Genus and Species: *Vitis vinifera*
	Native to the Mediterranean region and north into central Europe and the Middle East. Raisin grapes are most notably grown and dried in California, but also in other Mediterranean climates of Australia, Turkey, Greece, Iran and Chile.
Also called sultanas.	See www.sun-maid.com/en/recipes.html
	www.recipezaar.com/library/getentry.zsp?id=57

Exotic Prebiotic Foods

Exotic prebiotic foods are more difficult to locate, but are worth a try if you can find them. Some detective work may be needed to find them in stores or open markets.

Explore cookbooks and websites to find how to prepare them or to find recipes. To find out more about these more adventurous plants see Plants For A Future (www.pfaf.org/index.php). Search by the names of the genus and species.

Chicory root*	Family: *Asteraceae*
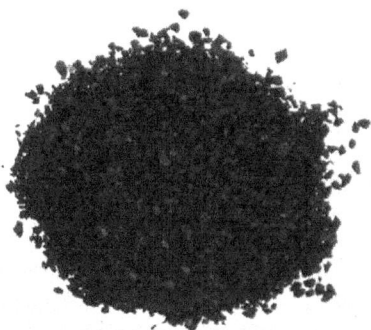	Genus and Species: *Cichorium intybus*
	Native to Europe. Grown in North America.
	Chicory is rich in inulin which often used as an ingredient in processed foods.
	The root is roasted and added to coffee in some cultures (New Orleans and parts of Europe).
	Note: Even though they do not have star status, try some of the greens that are chicory relatives. They include Belgian endive, radicchio, and curly endive.
Ground natural chicory	Order ground chicory at www.seedsofchange.com or www.orleanscoffee.com.

Burdock*	Season: Winter
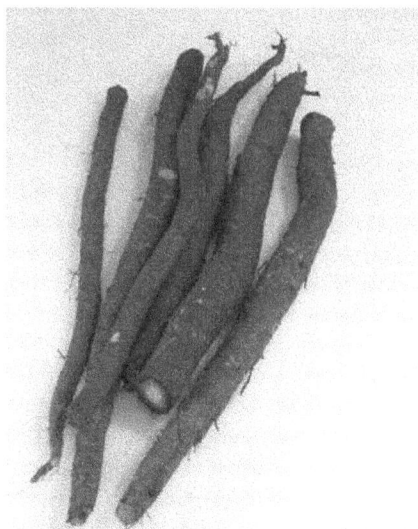	Family: *Asteraceae*
	Genus and Species: *Arctium lappa*
	Native to the Old World.
	Use gloves to prepare burdock because it stains your hands. Peel burdock root, and, if it is more than 1-inch-thick, halve lengthwise. Cut crosswise into 1-inch pieces. May also be julienned. Transfer burdock root to a bowl, then add 1 teaspoon vinegar and 2 cups water. Use in recipe of choice.
	About burdock www.asiafood.org/asianroots.cfm.
Also known as gobo.	Recipes www.prodigalgardens.info.

Dahlia tubers*	Season: August to October
[photo not available]	Family: *Asteraceae*
	Genus and Species: *Dahlia rosea*
	Native to Central America.
	Root of the flowering dahlia plant. The flowers are also edible. Uncommonly used as a food item. See www.pfaf.org/database/plants.php?Dahlia+rosea

Dandelion greens*	Season: Spring
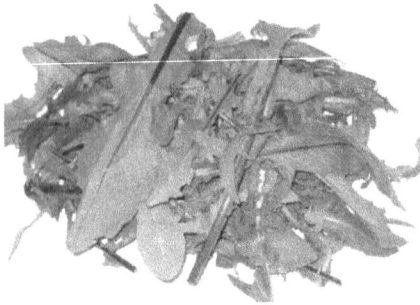	Native to Greece, cultivated throughout the world.
	Family: *Asteraceae*
	Genus and Species: *Taraxacum officinale*
	With a tart, bitter taste, dandelion greens may be steamed like other greens or used raw in a salad. Available from farmers markets.

Salsify, Purple*	Season: November-February (Year round)
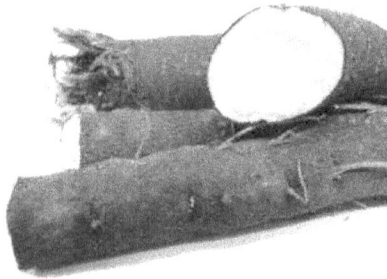	Family: *Asteraceae*
	Purple Genus and Species: *Tragopogon porrifolius*
	Black salsify, Scorzonera
	Genus and Species: *Scorzonera hispanica*
Photo source: Loves PLC www.lovesplc.co.uk	Native to Europe and Asia, grown in North America.
	Salsify must be prepped by scrubbing by the root, running it under cold water and then peeling it after cooking. If you chop or cut it before cooking, drop the cut pieces into acidulated water (vinegar or lemon juice added) to prevent discoloration. Use in recipe of choice.
Also called oyster plant.	See www.whatcom.wsu.edu/ag/homehort/plant/salsify.htm

Yacon* Photo source. UHTCO Corporation www.uhtco.ca	Family: *Asteraceae* Genus and Species: *Smallanthus sonchifolius* Native to the Andes Mountains. Recipes www.nicholsgardennursery.wordpress.com and search "Yacon." Also available in health food stores as a syrup for use as a sweetener.

Asteraceae Exotics

Many of the foods that are high in inulin and oligofructose are in the botanical family *Asteraceae*. Chicory, globe artichoke, Jerusalem artichoke, endive, dandelion greens, burdock or gobo root, salsify, and yacón are members of this family. While many of these vegetables are unfamiliar, they are beginning to appear at farmer's markets and supermarkets that carry more exotic produce. Yacón, for example, is made into a syrup that is advertised as being healthier for diabetics than sugar-based syrups.

Now that you are well versed on exotic produce, let's continue with all the rest of the prebiotic foods.

Prebiotic Foods – Everything Else

Wheat* Wheat berries, whole wheat flour. Cracked wheat bulgur.	When they are whole grain, these contain prebiotic fibers. Family: *Poaceae* Genus and Species: *Avena sativa* Native to southwestern Asia. Find whole grain flours for mail order at these web vendors www.bobsredmill.com www.kingarthurflour.com

Barley*	Family: *Poaceae*
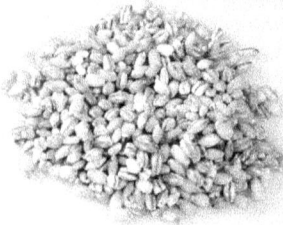	Genus and Species: *Avena sativa*
	Native to southwestern Asia, but grown in temperate climates all over the world.

Rye*	Family: *Poaceae*
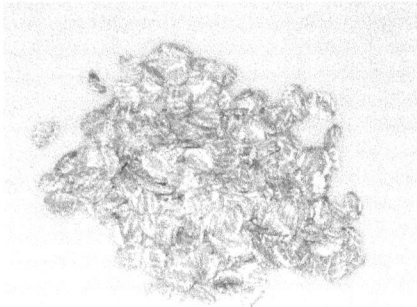	Genus and Species: *Avena sativa*
	Native to Turkey.

Oats	Contain the nondigestible fiber beta-glucan as well as phenols with antioxidant properties.
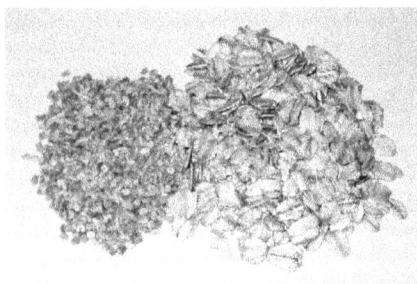	Family: *Poaceae*
	Genus and Species: *Avena sativa*
	Native to southwestern Asia, but cultivated throughout colder climates of Europe, North America, and Canada.
Steel cut oats, rolled oats	Find recipes at www.quakeroats.com

Dried beans, lentils and peas Legumes are a rich source of fiber and have other benefits.

Dried Beans

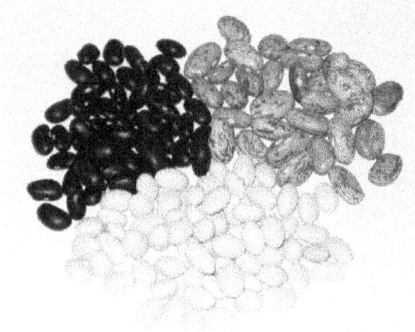

Availability: year round

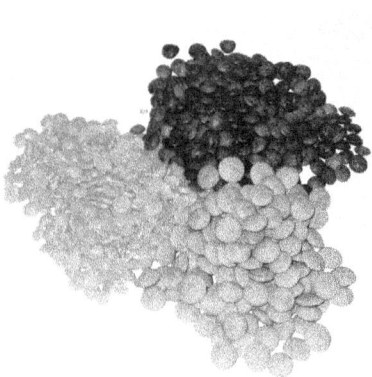

Family: *Fabaceae* (formerly *Leguminosae*)

About beans

www.pea-lentil.com/legumes.htm

www.beansforhealth.com/

www.foodsubs.com/Beans.html

www.fruitsandveggiesmatter.gov/month/beans.html

Recipes www.calbeans.com/recipes.html

www.bushbeans.com/recipes/recipes.php

Lentils

Family: *Fabaceae*

Genus and Species: *Lens culinaris*

Native to Mediterranean, western Asia.

Lentils have several subspecies that have different tastes and textures. They include green, red, French green, brown, and black beluga.

Chieftain® Wild Rice Company
www.chieftainwildrice.com/products/beans-lentils/lentils

Garbanzos, Ceci, Chickpeas

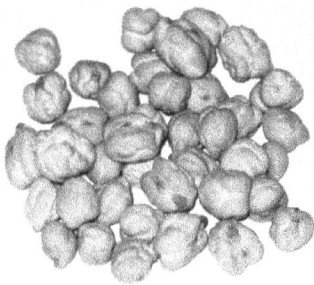

Family: *Fabaceae*

Genus and Species: *Cicer arietinum*

Available dried, canned and in hummus dips.

Native to western Asia.

Black eyed peas

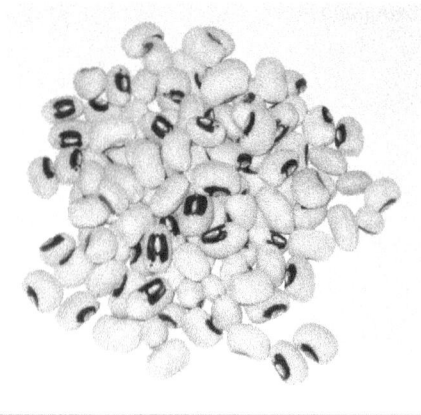

Family: *Fabaceae*

Vigna unguiculata unguiculata

Native to Africa.

Dried Peas

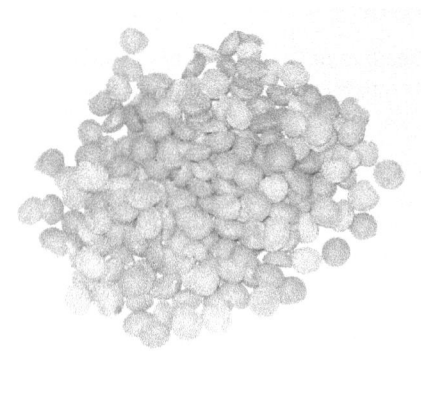

Family: *Fabaceae*

Genus and Species: *Pisum sativum*

Native to Southwest Asia.

Soybeans

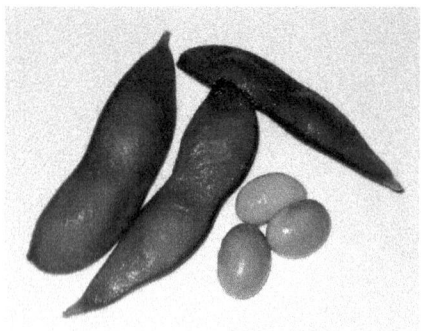

Family: *Fabaceae*

Genus and Species: *Glycine L. max (L.) Merr.*

Native to Asia.

Available as tofu, soymilk, edamame, and soy nuts.

Honey

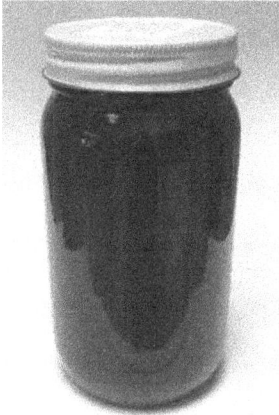

About honey: www.honey.com/consumers/

Recipes from the Honey Board, many use yogurt.
www.honey.com/consumers/recipes/recipes.asp

Note: "Do not feed a baby honey or syrup — at least for the first 6 months. Honey and syrups can contain spores of Clostridium botulinum. The immune systems of adults and older children can prevent the spores from growing once ingested. However, in an infant, these spores can grow and cause infant botulism." USDA

Flaxseed

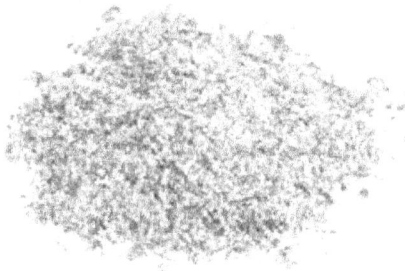

Family: *Linaceae*

Genus and Species: *Linum usitatissimum*

Native E. Mediterranean to India

Flaxseed is more digestible and bio-available when the seed is ground. It is available in well-stocked grocery stores in the baking section and can be purchased online. Because of the natural oils that tend to go rancid, flaxseed should be stored in the refrigerator.

Uses: Flaxseed is a great addition to yogurt at breakfast. Add 1 tablespoon to 8 ounces of yogurt. Try flax and honey as a toast topping. See more health information at www.mayoclinic.com/health/flaxseed/AN01258

Almonds

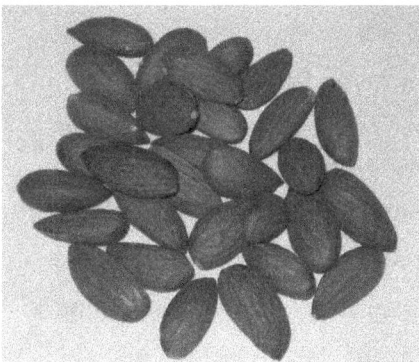

Family: *Rosaceae*

Genus and species: *Prunus dulcis*

Native to Southwestern Asia.

For more information, including recipes and storage tips, see www.almondsarein.com/AlmondLovers

Toss a few almonds on top of cereal in the morning or have ¼ cup as a snack.

Adding Prebiotic Foods to Your Culinary Repertoire

We have examples of what Josh, Ella, Kelly and Brittany have done to add prebiotic foods to their life. Since they have different home situations, lifestyles, and income levels, you may find that you identify with the Take-Out King, the Intrepid Eater, the Novice Cook, or the Health Nut. Their shopping needs, where they shop, where they find inspiration, and how they cook vary considerably.

The Take-Out King

Since Josh is single and is racking up his frequent flyer miles, he is the quintessential Take-Out King. His pantry is stocked with items that appeal to him, take little time to prepare, and come in packaging small enough that he does not waste food or begin growing molds and bacteria on leftover food in his refrigerator.

He prepares canned or dried soups for lunch or dinner when he is home. He keeps canned beans, canned beets, frozen peas, and frozen corn to make a simple salad. He keeps bread in the freezer to make a sandwich with peanut butter and banana or heats a frozen veggie burger in the microwave.

The deli counter is a great option for Josh, since he does not cook much and he can afford prepared take-out foods, which can be as expensive as a regular restaurant meal. He finds salads and vegetable side dishes that will counterbalance his on-the-go diet. Trying to keep sandwich meat fresh is a risky proposition unless he buys just what he can eat in a couple of days.

When Josh is on the go and eating out, he chooses vegetables and salads that he would be unlikely to eat at home. He has adapted and changed his diet by adding prebiotic vegetables, grains, and beans as well as other whole foods when he can find them. He will choose a salad bar or a vegetable soup when given the option.

Josh watches Iron Chef when he has the chance, although he would never consider cooking the way they do. He finds it exotic, but entertaining. Instead he prefers Mark Bittman's How to Cook Everything for its simple and straightforward recipes. He now enjoys a relaxed weekend evening cooking something simple for a woman friend and he buys an interesting salad or side dish from the gourmet deli counter. For inspiration he checks out www.recipes.com.

The Intrepid Eater

Ella, the Intrepid Eater, is always on the lookout for a new eating adventure and is not afraid to try exotic new foods and recipes. Her shopping varies by whether she is cooking only for herself or for her adult children when they visit her. Her pantry is the source of food in case her children drop by to see her.

On weekends she heads to the local farmers' market to pick up seasonal fruits and vegetables. She can get small amounts from the huge variety of produce. In her quest to add more exotic prebiotic foods to her diet, she first used some unusual greens that she steamed. Next, she roasted Jerusalem artichokes and later tried them in a soup with ginger and garlic. She then purchased chili peppers that she sautéed and enjoyed as an appetizer. Lastly, she tried Chinese winter melon that she used in an Asian-style soup.

Ella is a great cook and, because she has mild high blood pressure, she finds that cooking for herself helps her regulate her salt intake. When goes to the grocery store, she looks for high fiber foods like whole grain crackers and breads, grains that are used as savory side dishes like brown rice, bulgur, wild rice and whole grain couscous. She usually buys canned beans, but if her family is visiting, she will make a pot of beans using dried beans.

When she is looking for a culinary adventure, Ella checks out some favorite websites to get new ideas and research ingredients. She likes www.epicurious.com and the Post Punk Kitchen (www.theppk.com). When she is in the mood to watch a cooking show, she particularly likes *Lydia's Italian Table* on public television. Her new favorite cookbook is the *Moosewood Restaurant Cooks at Home* by Moosewood Collective.

Novice Cook

Kelly, the Novice Cook and college student, sticks with the supermarket for her shopping. She buys familiar produce including carrots, broccoli, and lettuce. She chooses fruit from whatever is in season that does not require more than a couple of minutes of preparation.

For lunch, she has a peanut butter sandwich and since meeting with the dietitian she chooses whole grain bread and peanut butter without added sugars or hydrogenated oils. She sometimes has soup and now chooses soups with beans and plenty of vegetables so that she can get a few more prebiotic foods into her diet. At dinnertime, she either eats alone or with her fiancé, Sean, and her effort varies according to her schedule. When Sean has dinner with her, she prepares pasta or a simple fish or chicken dish and Sean makes a salad. He will add prebiotic artichoke hearts and garbanzo beans to the salad.

Kelly watches Alton Brown's *Good Eats* and especially enjoys the shows on vegetables. She was pleased to know an answer on one of her biology test questions about bananas and ethylene gas. The answer came from an explanation Alton Brown offered on his show about how fruits ripen. Food and education at the same time! She is able to find some simple recipes that suit her cooking skills on Recipezaar (www.recipezaar.com).

The teenagers

Brittany, the Health Nut, shops for and feeds herself and hungry teenagers. She needs to go to the grocery store twice a week just to keep up with the demand for milk, bread, and bananas. She alternates between a conventional grocery store and Trader Joe's.

She chooses prepared cereal that is made from whole grains and buys lots, since her teenagers eat it for after school snacks as well as for breakfast. Her children are still picky about vegetables, but house rules require them to try any vegetable she serves. They do better with green salads, so she always has leaf lettuce, garbanzo beans, kidney beans, tomatoes, and salad dressing available.

She and her children take bag lunches to work and school. For these she alternates between sandwiches and leftovers from dinner that she reheats at work and that her children take in Thermos™ jars. Dinner is Brittany's opportunity to add some prebiotic grains and vegetables to her family's food offerings. The boys eat artichokes and asparagus with some parental encouragement.

She purchases lots of snacks for her teenagers who burn many calories in their sports activities. She always has popcorn on hand and she looks for cookies and crackers that are at least partly whole grain. Her teens are fond of tortilla chips (whole grain) and they eat them with hummus or quacamole.

Brittany makes an event of going to the farmers' market with friends on the weekend. They encourage each other to try new foods and share recipes and cooking tips about new foods. Recently she has added Jerusalem artichokes and kohlrabi to her repertoire.

Brittany watches *Americas Test Kitchen* and *Joanne Weir's Cooking Class*. She is inspired by the cookbooks: *Chez Panisse Vegetables* by Alice L. Waters and Molly Katzen's *The Vegetable Dishes I Can't Live Without.* She likes the Whole Foods website for information about vegetables and subscribes to EatingWell magazine and its email newsletters.

Recipes

Appetizers

Jicama at its Simplest

Peel jicama and slice into sticks. Use them as you would carrot sticks or celery but dipping into hummus or other dip.

Salads

Refrigerator Pickled Onions

> 4 large onions, peeled, sliced and separated into rings
> ½ C or more red wine vinegar to cover
> salt and pepper to taste

Toss all ingredients in a bowl. Store in a non-reactive glass or ceramic container in the refrigerator. This recipe takes about 5 minutes and gives you "pickled" onions in a few hours. They can be used in salads or on sandwiches and keep for several weeks. Sweet red onions work best.

Pantry Prebiotic Salad

> 1 can garbanzo beans or red kidney beans
> 1 jar artichoke hearts
> vinaigrette dressing

Mix together and serve.

Dandelion Green and Artichoke Salad

> ½ lb dandelion greens (2 cups)
> 2 C romaine lettuce
> ¼ C radishes trimmed and sliced
> 6 oz. marinated artichoke hearts

Use the artichoke marinade to make a dressing by adding:

> 1 T vinegar (red wine or balsamic)
> ¼ t Dijon mustard
> ½ t garlic minced
> salt and pepper to taste

Rinse, spin in a salad spinner, and trim the dandelion greens and lettuce. Add the radishes. Dress the salad. Arrange the artichokes on the top.

Soups

Jerusalem Artichoke Soup

> 1 lb Jerusalem artichokes
> 2 T olive oil
> 3 T grated ginger
> 3 cloves garlic minced
> 3 C chicken or vegetable stock
> salt and pepper to taste

Preheat a Dutch oven in a 350 degree oven. Scrub Jerusalem artichokes. Oven roast for 45 minutes. When fork tender, move to a food processor and process until smooth. Add ginger and garlic to the Dutch oven and sauté. Return puréed Jerusalem artichokes and add stock to the pan and warm through. Add seasonings. Garnish with a dollop of plain yogurt.

Vegetables

Slow Cooked Onions

> 4 large onions, peeled, sliced and separated into rings—red onions work well
> 3 T olive oil
> ½ t salt or 1 T Worcestershire sauce

Toss all ingredients in a bowl coating the onions with the liquid ingredients. Place in cast iron pot or oven-proof casserole in a 250 degree oven for 1 hour or in a slow cooker on high for 2 hours. Serve on sandwiches, as a pizza topping, or on French bread.

Oven Roasted Jerusalem Artichokes

> 1½ tablespoons olive oil
> 1½ pounds Jerusalem artichokes
> salt and freshly ground black pepper to taste

Preheat oven to 350 degrees F. Peel Jerusalem artichokes and slice into quarter inch pieces. Toss the Jerusalem artichokes, olive oil and salt and pepper in a bowl to coat. Transfer to a shallow roasting pan. Cook about 30 minutes (tossing once or twice) or until tender.

Pan Fried Jerusalem Artichokes

1½ lbs Jerusalem artichokes scrubbed and sliced thinly
4 T olive oil
Salt and pepper to taste
2 T minced parsley (optional)

Sauté sunchokes in a heavy frying pan over medium-high heat, stirring often, until they are browned lightly and tender (about 12 minutes).

Oven Roasted Leeks

2 large or 3 medium leeks (about 1½ lbs)
2 T olive oil
Salt and pepper to taste

Preheat oven to 350 degrees F. Trim, rinse and slice leeks. Place slices in a colander or salad spinner and rinse a second time to ensure that all of the sand is gone. Toss all ingredients in a bowl to coat the leeks with the oil. Move to an oven-proof casserole, cover, and bake 30 minutes.

Resources for Inspiration

When you are trying to eat well, inspiration plays a role in motivating you to try new foods and prepare them in new ways. You may get inspiration from several sources. When you go to a supermarket with a great produce section or a farmers' market, ask about foods that you have not seen before. The staff or the farmers will usually offer suggestions on how to prepare the food. Make a commitment to yourself to try a new food once a month. You need to repeat a recipe at least three times before it becomes a part of your regular repertoire. Use the new cookbook section at your local public library, quality television cooking shows, and internet sources for inspiration as well. When faced with a new vegetable or fruit, an internet search often provides the tip or recipe you need.

Websites we like for information about ingredients are

www.fruitsandveggiesmatter.gov/month/index.html

www.wholefoodsmarket.com/products/produce.php

Websites we like for recipes as well as the recipe sections of the two above are

www.eatingwell.com EatingWell is a also a magazine.

www.foodnetwork.com

www.epicurious.com Includes material from Gourmet and Bon Appetite magazines.

www.recipezaar.com

For really cutting-edge vegan fare, try www.theppk.com (the Post Punk Kitchen).

For an index of recipe websites, try www.foodieview.com.

What's Next?

To remind you why these foods are so important, the final chapter reviews the findings in the scientific literature that support the use of probiotics and prebiotics throughout the life cycle.

Chapter Ten: Probiotics and Prebiotics Through the Life Stages

Probiotics and prebiotics contribute to wellness by supporting digestive health and immunity throughout the life cycle.

Newborns and Infants

Early exposure to microbes takes place at birth. As discussed briefly in chapter one, early exposure is the basis for acquiring microbiota. The microbe exposure is primarily dependent upon two factors: the method of birth and the method of feeding. Natural birthing allows the fetus traveling down the birth canal to be exposed to their mother's natural microflora. When the infant is placed on the mother's breast, the newborn receives the mother's microflora which is contained in the mother's nipple and mammary gland ducts and is transferrred to the infant via breast milk. Thus breast milk is not sterile and each mother provides her own protective microflora to her infant. Breast milk also contains growth factors which foster the growth of certain species of bacteria such as those of the genus *Bifidobacteria*. Studies investigating breast milk have revealed that the profiles of the microflora differ between urban and rural areas, as well as parts of the world. These microbes colonize in the newborn's gastrointestinal tract where they begin to form a profile like a fingerprint. After weaning and towards the second year of age, a microbiota profile develops which characterizes an individual for life. The basic resident profile of microbes will remain the same and the individual's microbes will always revert back to that basic pattern. The factors thought to be influencing this profile or "fingerprint of microbes" include genetics and the environment.

When the birthing method is a Cesarean-section, the infant does not experience exposure to microbes in the birth canal and the newborn is essentially lifted out of the uterus in a sterile environment. Although exposed to the low levels of microbes contained in the placenta, amniotic fluid, and umbilical cord, the infant's microbiota development is delayed. The infant's microbiota development is influenced by the hospital environment and the use of antibiotics. The flora of an infant delivered by Cesarean-section or admitted into a nursery unit may more closely resemble that of the hospital environment than that of the mother.

When a newborn is breast-fed, it receives the mother's microbes. Additionally there may be an exchange process during breast-feeding when the infant's bacteria are exchanged with the mother's. When the infant receives sterile formula, the exposure is different. Although there is some transfer from the mother's skin and kisses, the fomula-fed newborn develops a different microbiota profile than that of the breast-fed infant. The bacterial colonization in early infancy in the breast-fed child is primarily of the genus *Bifidobacteria* as well as other genera like *Lactobacilli*.

Circumstances at birth (the method of delivery and the form of feeding) are of primary importance because these two factors are responsible for exposing the newborn to microbes that will colonize in their gut. A major role of the neonate's intestinal microbiota is to activate the mucosal immune system in the gut. What does that mean? It means that the microbiota provide a barrier effect to the lining of the gut that protects the newborn from harmful pathogens and allergenic substances. The presence of bacteria has a positive effect on the gut lining stimulating it to grow thicker which provides more more protection. In addition, bacteria communicate with and "train" the immune system cells present in the gut wall to respond appropriately resulting in local protection in the gut, as well as total body protection. This communication is called "cross-talk" and is the focus of a great deal of research attention.

The role and impact of the microbiota has been underestimated. Recently, as researchers uncover mechanisms for protection against diarrhea, malnutrition, inflammation, and gastrointestinal diseases, the tiny microbes are gaining new respect. Pregnant women and their physicians and mid-wives are beginning to understand the importance of vaginal delivery and breast-feeding which promote the exchange of microbial protection. Everyone is interested in the prevention of disease whether it is allergic disease, infectious disease, or the inflammatory response associated with the development of chronic disease. It is exciting to think that mothers can improve and ensure the future health of their children by their choice of delivery and feeding methods. Mothers should understand that the colonization of the gut of a vaginally-delivered, breast-fed infant resembles that of the mother. The role of the microbiotia is to protect the infant and contribute to the development of his or her immune system.

If an infant experiences inadequate colonization of microbiota and is raised and fed in a more sterile environment, it may put the infant at increased risk for digestive problems, including infections such as rotavirus (most comman intestinal virsus), allergy and autoimmune disease (for example, inflammatory bowel disease). The use of orally ingested probiotic bacteria, which affect gut immune response, is being considered for infants who may not have adequate colonization. Probiotics are specific bacteria which are safe and non-pathogenic, which when ingested regularly, provide a measurable benefit to the infant.

Some examples of onging research are summarized below.

Lactobacillus reuteri has been isolated in the digestive tract, the oral cavity, the stomach, small intestine, and colon as well as the vagina. Professor Gerhard Reuter has shown that *L. reuteri* is a bacterium that has its "natural ecological niche" in the digestive tract and that it is naturally established in the newborn child.

L. reuteri has been studied for the following uses:

- As a supplement during pregnancy

  Researchers have suggested providing probiotics to the mother during her pregnancy to influence the population of microflora to which the newborn is exposed in breast milk. A Swedish study demonstrated that the use of oral *Lactobacillus reuteri* during the last four weeks of pregnancy can exert effects beyond the gut wall — in this case mammary glands. Because it is found in the mammary gland, it is very likely the infant will receive the benefits of this bacteria while breast-feeding. More research is needed to show that the results are consistent and beneficial.

- As a supplement in breast-fed infants with colic

  The use of *L. reuteri* as a treatment for infantile colic in breast-fed infants was reported in a study conducted in Italy. Infantile colic is called the "mystery of infancy" and is very difficult to treat. In the Italian study the usual treatment with simethicone drops was compared to the use of the probiotic agent *L. reuteri*. They concluded that *L. reuteri* lessened the symptoms of colic in breast-fed infants within one week of treatment more effectively when compared with the usual treatment with simethicone. Additional studies are needed to examine the role of probiotics and to identify the ideal strain for treatment.

- As a supplement in mothers and infants to reduce allergy

  A reported study evaluated 188 families with allergic disease. Pregnant women received supplemental *L. reuteri* or placebo from week 36 of gestation until delivery. The babies then received the same product from birth to 12 months of age and were followed for another year. During this second year of testing the *L. reuteri* group had less eczema than the placebo group.

Infant Formulas with Probiotics and Prebiotics

Newborns fed infant formula have a different microflora profile than the breast-fed infant. Today probiotics have been added to some infant formulas. In the United States, Nestle Good Start® Natural Cultures™, a routine starter formula introduced in 2007 is the first formula with a probiotic, *Bifidobacterium lactis Bb 12*. It is a natural culture similar to those found in the digestive tract of breast-fed infants. *Bifidobacterium lactis Bb 12* is one of the most widely studied *bifidobacteria* which has been safely fed to infants and shows potential probiotic benefits. These include: increasing levels of *bifidobacteria* and secretory IgA (which plays a role in intestinal defense); reduction in the incidence and severity of acute diarrhea and in diarrhea in infants taking antibiotics; and reduction in the severity of allergic dermatitis.

With ingestion of a formula with *B. lactis Bb 12*, the microflora of the infant's gut changes. This is confirmed by examining the babies' stool. After seven days of ingesting *B. lactis Bb 12* the stool count of the bacteria reaches similar levels as that of the breast-fed infant. Stool pH shifts and the presence of short chain fatty acids confirm fermentation by the bacteria in the colon. As with all probiotic bacteria, their presence decreases once ingestion stops; so including them in formula or food is a desirable way to provide them to infants. Most importantly, *B. lactis* supplementation in both infants and young children has been associated with enhanced immunity. Studies demonstrated less fever, less frequency of antibiotic use, less otitis media infections, fewer sick days, and less rotaviral diarrhea with the use of *B lactis*. For mothers who cannot breast-feed or for those who want to transition to a formula Good Start® Natural Cultures™ offers a probiotic associated with enhanced immunity.

Infant formula manufacturers continue to look for ways to replicate the composition of human milk. Because human milk oligosaccharides (prebiotics) are thought to protect breast-fed infants by increasing *bifidobacteria*, studies were conducted in Europe and the United States which investigated the addition of galactooligosaccharides and fructooligosaccharides to infant formula. The studies demonstrated various outcomes including higher percentages of stool *bifidobacteria* and *lactobacilli*, increased fecal SIgA secretion (SIgA or secretory immunoglobulin A plays a significant role in gastrointestinal defense), decreased stool clostridia (thought to be bacterial pathogens), and softer stools more like breast-fed infants. Abbott Nutrition introduced Similac® Advance EarlyShield™ infant formula with prebiotics, to the United States in 2008. Because the addition of prebiotics results in softer stools, the infant should gradually transition to the formula, so their tolerance can be assessed. Adding prebiotics to infant formula may increase the amount of good bacteria in the digestive tract, however, more studies are needed to demonstrate this and other clinical benefits.

Young Children

Some of the best studies supporting a beneficial role for probiotics have been done in pediatric populations. Infants and children are very susceptible to exposure to pathogens which cause acute and persistent diarrhea. The benefits of probiotics use in this population include a reduction in the duration of acute diarrhea and a decrease in the incidence of diarrhea. The probiotics used in the studies included several strains of the species *B. lactis* and *L. rhamnosus*.

Antibiotic associated diarrhea is defined as an acute inflammation of the intestinal mucosa caused by the administration of the broad-spectrum antibiotics. The associated diarrhea is explained as a response to the disruption of the normal balance of the intestinal flora. Results of controlled trials that assessed over 750 children using either probiotics or placebo reduced the risk of diarrhea from 28% to 12% in the probiotic treatment group. The beneficial effects were strongest for *B. lactis* and *S. thermophilus*.

Results of a study in Australia have provided good news for working parents. Researchers found in their CUPDAY (Curtin University Probiotics in Day Care) Study that the use of their specially blended CUPDAY milk-based drink which contained the probiotic *Bifidobacterium lactis* (BL:CNCM 1-3446) along with a prebiotic blend which consisted of FOS and Acacia gum had a 20% reduction in the number of days the preschoolers experienced loose stools.This healthier outcome keeps children in preschool and means that parents need not miss work to care for them.

As a dietitian, I recommend that parents begin feedings of naturally fermented foods during the introduction of solids. And when a child does undergo antibiotic therapy, it is important to daily replenish their gut microbiota with foods containing the live cultures of beneficial microbes. Probiotic foods should be given at a different time from the antibiotics, since antibiotics destroy probiotic bacteria.

Children and Yogurt

Children will accept the taste of plain yogurt if it's introduced with their first foods. Later when they discover the flavored versions, they will naturally prefer them for sweeter taste. They will still accept the plain as a topping for fresh fruits and as a side for dipping because it is a familiar taste. Plus you can always sweeten the plain yogurt with fresh fruit pureed or jams. To assure that you are getting live active cultures look for the live active culture seal.

Children and Kefir

Kefir flavored with various fruits is acceptable to children as a beverage. Getting a child to accept a plain kefir is more difficult. Its sour taste is due to the live cultures it contains. Mix 2 ounces of kefir and 2 ounces of fresh juice and enjoy it with them. Serve frequently as familiarity brings acceptance of foods with new tastes.

Supplements

Chapter two discusses food and beverage products that are naturally fermented and contain live cultures. I do not recommend parents experiment on their own with supplements of probiotics, because there are just too many unanswered questions regarding safety. If you want to use a supplement, check with your physician for guidance and ask about adverse effects resulting from their use.

Allergic Disorders

Allergic conditions are increasing in the United States at distressing rates. Because many scientists believe an allergic response to be related to an excessive or imbalanced immune response, probiotics are being extensively studied, not only for prevention, but also for the reduction of symptoms of allergic diseases. Studies with infants and children have resulted in the most positive findings.

Atopic eczema, whose symptoms include an itchy, scaly red rash, usually begins early in life and is particularly distressing for infants and young children. It is considered to be an early manifestation of allergy as half of the children with a history of eczema go on to develop other allergic conditions such as asthma. Researchers report there are distinct differences in the *bifidobacteria* microbiota in infants who later develop atopic disease when compared to healthy infants. In the allergic child they have found lower levels of *bifidobacteria* as well as lower levels of lactic acid bacteria.

Breast-fed infants have a lower incidence of eczema. The microbiota development of the breast-fed infant is being extensively studied. For example, at Stanford University mothers of breast-fed babies provided their babies stools for analysis over the first year of life. The researchers found that each baby had different microbes colonizing its gut at different stages. The goal of the study was to examine what occurs in the healthy breast fed infant.

Can researchers simulate the breast milk microbiota by providing probiotics and prebiotics to the non breast-fed infant? Until that question is answered, it is best to trust Mother Nature and promote breast-feeding during that first year.

However, if breast-feeding is not possible, there may be benefit in using probiotics to modify the gut's microbiota. Researchers have investigated the effectiveness of various strains of probiotics and there have been some favorable outcomes in some allergic conditions in infants and children both for the prevention of disease and for the improvement of symptoms. And there have been some positive results in controlled trials where the researchers found that *L. rhamnosus GG* and *B. lactis* were effective in improving skin conditions caused by eczema. Other studies have demonstrated that *Lactobacillus GG* may reduce the eczema flare-ups in toddlers.

One theory for the increase in allergic disease is that we do not get the early exposure to bacteria that our ancestors got before our food became so clean. The premise is that it takes early exposure to bacteria to stimulate an immune response. The inflammatory response is thought to actually prevent allergies. This idea that allergic disease has increased due to lack of early stimulation is of great interest to researchers.

A recent study examined the effects of giving probiotics to pregnant women in their eighth month of pregnancy who had a history of allergies. They then provided the same probiotics to their infants for six months. When their infants were compared to the non-treated control infants from mother's who did not receive probiotics, the group of infants who did receive probiotics was 30% less likely to develop atopic eczema.

So the best advice to mothers who are concerned about allergic diseases is to breast-feed and, if that is not possible, to consult with the child's pediatrician about the potential use of infant formulas containing probiotics.

Older Children and Adolescents with Constipation

Digestive illness or dysfunction are common to all age groups. Constipation can occur in older children and adolescents. With constipation there is incomplete stool evacuation. This is often referred to as irregularity. You may be thinking "what is irregularity?" We describe our lower or large bowel and its colon's function with the term "regular" meaning bowel movements occur without straining, with complete evacuation, and on a regular basis. There is a bell shaped curve of how often per day or per week they occur, however, for good digestive health a bowel movement each day is ideal. Although every two to three days is normal, if evacuation is complete. As a pediatric dietitian, I have treated a lot of constipated children and adolescents. These normal children were suffering from constipation secondary to either "withholding" bowel movements or their diets were terribly constipating (meaning they ate few whole fresh foods). In fact, many had to have frequent "clean outs" of stool until their colon regained its normal size having expanded due to holding so much stool. Once the colon was normal size, we could treat them with diet, fiber, fermented products, and fluids.

Once treated for constipation, children and adolescents, who have healthy whole foods and a serving of yogurt with live active cultures on a daily basis should be regular. If not, try specialty yogurts and cheeses to improve regularity. You just have to try each one on a regular basis (usually daily for two weeks) to see if you get positive results. Be aware that these products may not have been studied in children.

We look at our children's stool from infancy through childhood and then privacy takes over. However, for good digestive health you should look at your stools as an indicator of how well your body and your GI tract are functioning. It is one of the few things originating in our bodies that we can actually examine as an indicator of good or poor health. So start looking at your stool. The accompanying box provides vivid descriptions.

Stool Gazing

Looking at and evaluating one's bowel movements, commonly known as stools, for consistency, shape and color can be very insightful and revealing as you evaluate your overall health. The body has a natural process for the elimination of its wastes. We tend to examine everything else to give us an indication of our health status. We look at the condition of our skin, eyes, hair, teeth, and mouth so why not examine the stool? The following guide provides descriptions of problematic stools based on consistency, shape, and color. Probable causes and therapies are listed. You may have an indicator in your stool of a serious condition which requires a physician's expertise.

For comparison, the model stool is described, which ideally, should be what you are striving for.

Model Stool is bulky, soft, and easy to pass with a uniform shape (torpedo like).

Consistency

Hard stools	Hard and difficult to pass (may be small separate pellets or lumped together).
Possible causes	Slow transit time — the stool is moving too slowly and becomes drier as fluid is absorbed.
	Lack of fiber results in a dry stool (fiber retains fluid).
	Low carbohydrate diet (proteins and fats do not contain fiber).
Cures	Increase fluids, especially water
	Add fiber — wheat bran (will absorb water and add bulk to the stool)
	Increase raw fruits and vegetables which contribute natural fluid and fiber.
	Alter transit time — try specialty yogurts.

Too soft	Liquid stools which move very rapidly and sometimes with great urgency
Possible causes	Rapid transit time (little fluid being absorbed along the way). (The GI tract handles about eight liters of fluid provided for digestion and ease of transport each day. If the contents are moving too rapidly, the fluid is not absorbed). Changes in diet (increase in fiber or raw foods which contribute fluid and indigestible material to the stool). Pathogens (bacterial or viral infections can result in soft watery stools as your GI tract tries to rid the body of these harmful organisms).
Cures	Eat a diet without raw foods and visible fibers. Cook your foods and chew thoroughly so they are easier to digest. See an MD for treatment of your infection or suggestion of medications to slow transit time.

Stool Gazing Alerts

Skinny stools	This is an alert for something that is abnormal in the colon and the only way the stool can pass is in a very thin form. It could mean polyps or a mass in the colon. See an MD for evaluation.
Floating stools	Stools are not supposed to float on water. If they do, you may well be excreting fat in your stools which means you are not digesting and absorbing it. Floating stools with fat have such a strong odor the entire house might smell. So unless you are eating foods with Olestra (an indigestible fat substitute) or taking a medication for weight loss that causes you not to absorb all the fats you eat, you should see your doctor.
Black stools	May be due to the supplements you are taking (e.g. iron). Stop the supplement for a while to see if the color changes. Or there could be bleeding in the upper intestinal tract (the esophagus) due to reflux which can damage the lining of the esophagus, or the bleeding may be in the stomach. You need to see an MD.

Green stools	If you are eating or drinking foods with green coloring or naturally green foods that can be the cause. If you are not eating green foods, but you are taking iron, the iron could be the culprit. If none of the above are true and you also have loose stools, it may be that bile excreted from the liver is not breaking down. You should see a physician.
Gray stools	May be caused by medications (e.g. anti-diarrheal medications). Or it could be a lack of bile (excreted by the liver and necessary for the digestion of fats). If you see this type of stool and are not taking an anti-diarrheal medication, see an MD.
Red stools	May be related to something you ate with red food coloring (candies or drinks) or a food that is naturally red such as red beets. If you have not eaten red foods possibly you are bleeding from hemorrhoids (internal or external) or you could have something more serious, so seek medical care.
Yellow stools	May be associated with floating stools and excess fat in the stool. It could be a sign of a serious malabsorption disorder meaning you are not digesting and absorbing your food. If this is the case, you should see your doctor. Yellow stools are normal in breast-fed infants.

Pregnant Women

Digestive "ills" are very familiar to pregnant women. Hormonal changes influence her GI tract and as the growing fetus competes for space the pregnant woman confronts nausea, reflux, constipation, and gas. All of these separately, but certainly in combination, can be responsible for great discomfort.

Eating foods with live active cultures on a daily basis may well quell these symptoms common to pregnancy. It is wise to use fermented soy or dairy products with probiotics, particularly the plain yogurts and kefir. In addition, the prebiotics contained in these foods are particularly valuable in pregnancy to keep the beneficial microbial residents flourishing in the pregnant woman's colon. When there is a good balance between probiotics and prebiotics, regularity is enhanced, the nutrient value of the diet is improved, and she will suffer less from reflux and gas. Plus, you will have a healthful microbiotia for transfer to your baby at birth.

If constipated, the pregnant woman may want to try some of the specialty yogurts designed to enhance regularity. She should try eating specialty yogurt daily and see if there is a difference after ten to fourteen days. In addition the specialty cheeses may have a role in the pregnant woman's diet. Cheese, although delicious and nutritious, does not contribute fluids or fiber or even any significant amount of the fermentable microbes that are used in making aged cheeses. However, the specialty cheeses are designed to contribute live cultures for regularity and there are products with the prebiotic inulin. The cheeses and some of the other specialty products for example cereals, juices, and bars with probiotics and prebiotics are good options for pregnancy.

Adult Women

Women may experience vaginal infections. Normally, *lactobacillus* strains are the usual inhabitants of the vaginal tract. However, infections do result from the migration of microbes contained in the colon and stool. More frequently in the past, but sometimes, women used yogurt douches with the addition of *lactobacillus* strains to repopulate the vaginal tract. Today the research is concentrating on the potential of probiotic use to treat or improve the outcome of women who suffer from bacterial or yeast infections. Some studies show positive results with orally administered *lactobacillus* strains, as they do pass through the GI tract and migrate to the vaginal tract where they restore the healthy vaginal flora. Another study used yogurt as the means of delivery and demonstrated improvement. However, not all studies showed positive outcomes. So the research continues.

Lactose Intolerance

Lactose intolerance occurs in individuals who have low levels of the intestinal enzyme lactase that digests lactose (milk sugar). It affects children, teens, adults, and the older generation. Lactose intolerance can also be transient due to severe injury to the wall of the GI tract caused by infection and inflammation as injury can result in less enzyme production. The symptoms are not pretty with maldigestion resulting in lower abdominal pain, discomfort, and gas. In addition these symptoms may be accompanied by explosive diarrhea.

Individuals with lactose intolerance can generally tolerate yogurt with live cultures mainly because the starter cultures (*Streptococcus thermophilus* and *Lactobacillus delbrueckii* subsp *bulgaricus*) used in yogurt release lactase in the small bowel where it aids the digestion of lactose. If you suspect lactose intolerance, try eliminating all milk products to see if your symptoms resolve. Then try adding back small amounts of yogurt (3-4 tablespoons) with the above starter cultures as you test for tolerance. You should be symptom free. If you are not symptom free, you can always use soy yogurt with live cultures, which is lactose free since it does not contain cow's milk.

Older Adults

Constipation

In older adults there seems to be a natural slowing of the GI tract and its function. This slowdown of GI function is normal with age. Some people notice as they get older that it takes longer to digest a meal. Reflux may appear, accompanied by discomfort and a burning in the throat and constipation becomes more the norm than the exception. Regularity requires daily attention to diet. As with any age, a diet of natural foods with whole grains, fruits, vegetables, beans, peas, and nuts provides fiber and **prebiotic potentials**. In addition, fluid plays a role in hydrating the body and contributing to a softer stool. But older people just seem to need a little help. So rather than take stool softeners, over the counter laxatives, or fiber supplements, try probiotics taken in a nutritious food that influences bowel transit time.

Bowel transit time is the amount of time it takes for ingested food to travel through your GI tract and pass out as stool. Normally it is anywhere from 45-72 hours with the majority of the time spent in the colon. Many things can influence or alter an individual's transit time including diet composition, stress, activity, medications, and age. Many older adults are less mobile and possibly on medications (such as antidepressants and blood pressure medications) that can slow down the GI tract.

In studies, some probiotic strains have been studied and some strains (such as *Bifidobacterium animalis DN-173010*) when added to fermented milk and taken two to three times a day was effective in decreasing bowel transit time. I have recommended the use of a specialty yogurt with a blend of microbes including *Bifidobacterium animalis DN-173 010*. My clients report they can experience daily bowel movements.

Older adults may eat a lot of cheese, since it is convenient and nutritious. But because cheese can contribute to constipation, I advise them to try the cheeses with live active probiotics. Research shows that such cheeses decrease transit time. You might try one of them daily for two weeks and see if you notice a difference.

Diarrhea

Diarrhea can also be a frequent occurrence in older people. Acute (less than two weeks) and chronic (thirty days or more) infectious diarrhea can be life threatening. Diarrhea can also be caused by abnormalities of digestive function such as lactose intolerance, gluten intolerance, or pancreatic abnormalities. The frequent ingestion of sugarless candies with nondigestible carbohydrates can cause diarrhea. Probiotics will often help minimize the diarrhea.

Infectious diarrhea in the elderly can quickly lead to dehydration and electrolyte abnormalities. It is imperative to prevent infectious causes immediately. Drinks containing probiotics have been shown to minimize the diarrhea among older people who are taking antibiotics. The findings of this study are specific to a product with a unique strain *Lactobacillus casei DN-114 001*.

Immunity

People over 60 years of age are candidates for probiotic containing foods and beverages primarily due to the decline in the immune system that makes them less able to defend against infections. Scientists theorize that this population has less of the friendly bacteria in their gut than younger people. By replacing this loss with products full of protective bacteria, the hope is that immunity in this population will be improved. When studies have demonstrated enough positive findings, we will find it more common to give fortified probiotic food and drinks to older people especially those hospitalized, in long term care, or when they are at greater risk for incurring an infection.

Irritable Bowel Syndrome (IBS)

Irritable bowel can affect all age groups. It is difficult to define and usually means complaints of intermittent bloating, gas, pain, diarrhea, and constipation. Similar symptoms after a bout of infection are known as post-infectious irritable bowel syndrome. Studies using the animal model have shown promising roles for probiotics. In humans, probiotics have been used to reduce the duration of an acute infection.

For adults with IBS Procter and Gamble has made the probiotic supplement Align® with *Bifidobacterium infantis 35624*, which seems to help people. Although this book focuses on food for probiotic and prebiotic sources, this supplement is produced with P&G's quality control and supporting research studies. However, as always we recommend you discuss probiotic supplements with your physician.

Conclusion

This summary is just a small part of the research findings and potential opportunities involving the use of probiotics and their important role in health. Future research is expected to reveal ways to reduce illness and its symptoms as well as prevent future illnesses. How will these tiny microbes be provided?

There will be products for all age groups — some designed for target populations such as pregnant women and older adults. Enhanced immunity is expected to be the most consistent driving force. There is interesting research on the horizon exploring whether the gut's microbiota mix can influence regulation of appetite, glycemic control, and body weight.

Appendices, References and Resources

Appendices

See website www.gutinsight.com

References and Resources

Chapter One

Baker M. Man's best friend. New take on infection-causing bugs. Stanford Medicine Magazine Summer 2006. http://stanmed.stanford.edu/2006summer/bacteria.html

FAO/WHO. The Food and Agriculture Organization of the United Nations and the World Health Organization Joint FAO/WHO expert consultation on evaluation of health and nutritional properties of probiotics in food including powder milk with live lactic acid bacteria. 10-1-2001. 2001. http://www.who.int/entity/foodsafety/publications/fs_management/en/probiotics.pdf

Douglas LE, Sanders ME. Probiotics and Prebiotics in Dietetics Practice JADA. Volume 108, Issue 3, Pages 510-521 (March 2008)

Guarner F. Enteric flora in health and disease. Digestion. 2006;73 Suppl 1:5-12.

Huffnagle G, Wenick S. The Probiotics Revolution: The Definitive guide to safe, natural health solutions using probiotic and prebiotic foods and supplements. NY, NY: Bantam, 2007.

Lu L, Walker WA. Pathologic and physiologic interactions of bacteria with the gastrointestinal epithelium. Am J Clin Nutr. 2001 Jun;73(6):1124S-1130S.

Metchnikoff E. The prolongation of life—optimistic studies. London: Heinemann, 1908.

National Center for Complementary and Alternative Medicine (NCCAM) An Introduction to probiotics. http://nccam.nih.gov/health/probiotics/index.htm

Probiotics: Their Potential to Impact Human Health addresses the biological processes and physiological benefits of probiotics. CAST Issue Paper Number 36 October 2007. www.cast-science.org

Reid R. So, which bacteria did you eat today? 2005, Danone Vitapole DVD video.

Sanders ME. Probiotics: considerations for human health. Nutr Rev. 2003 Mar;61(3):91-9. Review.

Schrezenmeir J, de Vrese M. Probiotics, prebiotics, and synbiotics— approaching a definition. Am J Clin Nutr. 2001 Feb;73(2 Suppl):361S-364S.

Simpson S, Ash C, Pennisi E, Travis J. The Gut: Inside Out. Science 25 March 2005: Vol. 307. no. 5717, p. 1895

Turnbaugh PJ, Ley RE, Mahowald MA, Magrini V, Mardis ER, Gordon JI. An obesity-associated gut microbiome with increased capacity for energy harvest. Nature. 2006 Dec 21;444(7122):1027-31.

Chapter Two

Bamforth, CW. Food, fermentation and micro-organisms. Oxford: Blackwell, 2005.

Davidson RH, Duncan SE, Hackney CR, Eigel WN, Boling JW. Probiotic culture survival and implications in fermented frozen yogurt characteristics. J Dairy Sci. 2000 Apr;83(4):666-73.

Duggan C, Gannon J, Walker WA. Protective nutrients and functional foods for the gastrointestinal tract. Am J Clin Nutr. 2002 May;75(5):789-808.

FAO/WHO. The Food and Agriculture Organization of the United Nations and the World Health Organization Joint FAO/WHO expert consultation on evaluation of health and nutritional properties of probiotics in food including powder milk with live lactic acid bacteria. 10-1-2001. http://www.who.int/entity/foodsafety/publications/fs_management/en/probiotics.pdf

FAO/WHO. Guidelines for the Evaluation of Probiotics in Food. Report of a Joint FAO/WHO Working Group on Drafting Guidelines for the Evaluation of Probiotics in Food. London Ontario, Canada , April 30 and May 1, 2002 http://www.who.int/foodsafety/fs_management/en/probiotic_guidelines.pdf

Farnworth ER, Mainville I, Desjardins MP, Gardner N, Fliss I, Champagne C. Growth of probiotic bacteria and bifidobacteria in a soy yogurt formulation. Int J Food Microbiol. 2007 May 1;116(1):174-81.

Guarner F. Enteric flora in health and disease. Digestion. 2006;73 Suppl 1:5-12.

Hekmat S, McMahon DJ. Survival of Lactobacillus acidophilus and Bifidobacterium bifidum in ice cream for use as a probiotic food. J Dairy Sci. 1992 Jun;75(6):1415-22.

IFIC. Functional Foods Fact Sheet: Probiotics and Prebiotics. http://www.ific.org/publications/factsheets/preprobioticsfs.cfm

Koebnick C, Wagner I, Leitzmann P, Stern U, Zunft HJ. Probiotic beverage containing Lactobacillus casei Shirota improves gastrointestinal symptoms in patients with chronic constipation. Can J Gastroenterol. 2003 Nov;17(11):655-9.

McGee, Harold. On Food and Cooking: The Science and Lore of the Kitchen. New York: Scribner, 2004.

National Center for Complementary and Alternative Medicine (NCCAM) An Introduction to probiotics. http://nccam.nih.gov/health/probiotics/index.htm

Sanders ME. Dairy & Food Culture Technologies. http://www.mesanders.com

Sanders ME. Probiotics: considerations for human health. Nutr Rev. 2003 Mar;61(3):91-9. Review.

Simpson S, Ash C, Pennisi E, Travis J . The Gut: Inside Out. Science 25 March 2005: Vol. 307. no. 5717, p. 1895.

Chapter Three

American Institute for Cancer Research. Moving Toward a Plant-Based Diet.
http://www.aicr.org/site/PageServer?pagename=pub_plant_based_diet

Camire ME, Dougherty MP. Raisin dietary fiber composition and in vitro bile acid binding. J Agric Food Chem. 2003 Jan 29;51(3):834-7.

Cummings JH, Macfarlane GT, Englyst HN. Prebiotic digestion and fermentation. Am J Clin Nutr. 2001 Feb;73(2 Suppl):415S-420S.

Diaz-Rubio ME, Saura-Calixto F. Dietary fiber in brewed coffee. J Agric Food Chem. 2007 Mar 7;55(5):1999-2003. Epub 2007 Feb 13.

Dietary Reference Intakes for Energy, Carbohydrate, Fiber, Fat, Fatty Acids, Cholesterol, Protein, and Amino Acids (Macronutrients) (2005) National Academy of Sciences. Institute of Medicine. Food and Nutrition Board. Chapter 7 - Dietary, Functional, and Total Fiber.

Fraser GE, Bennett HW, Jaceldo KB, Sabate J. Effect on body weight of a free 76 Kilojoule (320 calorie) daily supplement of almonds for six months.J Am Coll Nutr. 2002 Jun;21(3):275-83.

Gibson GR, McCartney AL, Rastall RA. Prebiotics and resistance to gastrointestinal infections. Br J Nutr. 2005 Apr;93 Suppl 1:S31-4.

Gibson GR, Roberfroid MB. Dietary modulation of the human colonic microbiota: introducing the concept of prebiotics. J Nutr. 1995 Jun;125(6):1401-12.

Gibson GR. Dietary modulation of the human gut microflora using prebiotics. Br J Nutr. 1998 Oct;80(4):S209-12.

Gibson, Glenn R; Roberfroid, MB. Handbook of prebiotics. Boca Raton : CRC Press, c2008.

Gibson, Glenn R; Rastall, Robert. Prebiotics : development & application. Chichester, England ; Hoboken, NJ : John Wiley & Sons, c2006.

Gibson GR. Dietary modulation of the human gut microflora using the prebiotics oligofructose and inulin. J Nutr. 1999 Jul;129(7 Suppl):1438S-41S.

Griffin IJ, Abrams SA. Methodological considerations in measuring human calcium absorption: relevance to study the effects of inulin-type fructans. Br J Nutr. 93(Suppl 1):S105-110, 2005.

Hughes SA, Shewry PR, Gibson GR, McCleary BV, Rastall RA. In vitro fermentation of oat and barley derived beta-glucans by human faecal microbiota. FEMS Microbiol Ecol. 2008 Jun;64(3):482-93.

IOM. Dietary Reference Intakes: Proposed Definition of Dietary Fiber (2001) Institute of Medicine

Kaur N, Gupta AK. Applications of inulin and oligofructose in health and nutrition. J Biosci. 2002 Dec;27(7):703-14.

Kolida S, Gibson GR. Prebiotic capacity of inulin-type fructans. J Nutr. 2007 Nov;137(11 Suppl):2503S-2506S.

Landow MV. Trends in dietary carbohydrates research. New York : Nova Science Publishers, c2006.

Lee HC. Jenner AM. Low CS. Lee YK. Effect of tea phenolics and their aromatic fecal bacterial metabolites on intestinal microbiota. Research in Microbiology. 157(9):876-84, 2006 Nov.

Lomax AR, Calder PC. Prebiotics, immune function, infection and inflammation: a review of the evidence. Br J Nutr. 2008 Sep 25:1-26.

Mandalari G, Nueno-Palop C, Bisignano G, Wickham MS, Narbad A. Investigation of the potential prebiotic properties of almond (Amygdalus communis L.) seeds. Appl Environ Microbiol. 2008 May 23.

McGee, Harold. On Food and Cooking: The Science and Lore of the Kitchen (2004)

Merck Manual Online. Gas-Related Complaints. http://www.merck.com/mmpe/sec02/ch008/ch008d.html#

Moshfegh AJ, Friday JE, Goldman JP, Ahuja JK. Presence of inulin and oligofructose in the diets of Americans. J Nutr. 1999 Jul;129(7 Suppl):1407S-11S.

Pereira DI, Gibson GR.Effects of consumption of probiotics and prebiotics on serum lipid levels in humans. Crit Rev Biochem Mol Biol. 2002;37(4):259-81

Roberfroid M. Prebiotics: the concept revisited. J Nutr. 2007 Mar;137(3 Suppl 2):830S-7S.

Roy CC, Kien CL, Bouthillier L, Levy E. Short-chain fatty acids: ready for prime time? Nutr Clin Pract. 2006 Aug;21(4):351-66.

Sanz ML, Polemis N, Morales V, Corzo N, Drakoularakou A, Gibson GR, Rastall RA. In vitro investigation into the potential Prebiotic activity of honey oligosaccharides. J Agric Food Chem. 2005 Apr 20;53(8):2914-21.

Seeram NP. Berry fruits for cancer prevention: current status and future prospects. J Agric Food Chem. 2008 Feb 13;56(3):630-5. Epub 2008 Jan 23.

Stevenson DG, Jane JL, Inglett GE. Characterisation of Jicama (Mexican potato) (Pachyrhizus erosus L. Urban) starch from taproots grown in USA and Mexico. Source: STARCH-STARKE Volume: 59 Issue: 3-4 Pages: 132-140 Published: MAR 2007

Swennen K. Courtin CM. Delcour JA. Non-digestible oligosaccharides with prebiotic properties. Critical Reviews in Food Science & Nutrition. 46(6):459-71, 2006.

Tannock, GW. Probiotics and prebiotics: scientific aspects. Wymondham : Caister Academic Press, c2005.

Tannock, GW. Probiotics and prebiotics: where are we going? Norfolk, England : Caister Academic Press, c2002.

Van Loo J, Coussement P, de Leenheer L, Hoebregs H, Smits G. On the presence of inulin and oligofructose as natural ingredients in the western diet. Crit Rev Food Sci Nutr. 1995 Nov;35(6):525-52

Van Loo JA. Prebiotics promote good health: the basis, the potential, and the emerging evidence. J Clin Gastroenterol. 2004 Jul;38(6 Suppl):S70-5.

Willett WC. Diet and health: what should we eat? Science. 1994 Apr 22;264(5158):532-7.

Prebiotics and Probiotics - Ingredients Handbook. Leatherhead Food International. January 1, 2000.

Chapter Four

Bouhnik Y, Raskine L, Simoneau G, Vicaut E, Neut C, Flourié B, Brouns F, Bornet FR. The capacity of nondigestible carbohydrates to stimulate fecal bifidobacteria in healthy humans: a double-blind, randomized, placebo-controlled, parallel-group, dose-response relation study. Am J Clin Nutr. 2004 Dec;80(6):1658-64.

Dietary Reference Intakes for Energy, Carbohydrate, Fiber, Fat, Fatty Acids, Cholesterol, Protein, and Amino Acids (Macronutrients) (2005) National Academy of Sciences. Institute of Medicine. Food and Nutrition Board. Chapter 7 - Dietary, Functional, and Total Fiber (PDF|514 KB)

Gibson GR. Prebiotics as gut microflora management tools. J Clin Gastroenterol. 2008 Jul;42 Suppl 2:S75-9.

Griffin IJ, Abrams SA. Methodological considerations in measuring human calcium absorption: relevance to study the effects of inulin-type fructans. Br J Nutr. 93(Suppl 1):S105-110, 2005.

Jones PJ. Clinical nutrition: 7. Functional foods--more than just nutrition. CMAJ. 2002 Jun 11;166(12):1555-63.

Redgwell RJ, Fischer M. Dietary fiber as a versatile food component: an industrial perspective. Mol Nutr Food Res. 2005 Jun;49(6):521-35.

Roberfroid MB. Inulin-type fructans: functional food ingredients. J Nutr. 2007 Nov;137(11 Suppl):2493S-2502S.

Roberfroid MB. Functional food concept and its application to prebiotics. Dig Liver Dis. 2002 Sep;34 Suppl 2:S105-10.

Roberfroid MB. Concepts in functional foods: the case of inulin and oligofructose. J Nutr. 1999 Jul;129(7 Suppl):1398S-401S.

Roberfroid MB. Prebiotics and synbiotics: concepts and nutritional properties. Br J Nutr. 1998 Oct;80(4):S197-202.

Saulnier DM, Gibson GR, Kolida S. In vitro effects of selected synbiotics on the human faecal microbiota composition. FEMS Microbiol Ecol. 2008 Jul 30.

Scholz-Ahrens KE, Ade P, Marten B, Weber P, Timm W, Asil Y, Gluer CC, Schrezenmeir J. Prebiotics, probiotics, and synbiotics affect mineral absorption, bone mineral content, and bone structure. J Nutr. 2007 Mar;137(3 Suppl 2):838S-46S.

Tharanathan, R. Starch - Value Addition by Modification. Critical Reviews in Food Science & Nutrition; Jul/Aug 2005, Vol. 45 Issue 5, p371-384

Vonk RJ, Hagedoorn RE, de Graaff R, Elzinga H, Tabak S, Yang YX, Stellaard F. Digestion of so-called resistant starch sources in the human small intestine. Am J Clin Nutr. 2000 Aug;72(2):432-8.

Chapter Five

Centers for Disease Control and Prevention. Bad bug book: foodborne pathogenic microorganisms and natural toxins handbook http://vm.cfsan.fda.gov/~mow/intro.html

Centers for Disease Control and Prevention. FAQ on foodborne illness. Index of U.S. government sites related to food safety http://www.foodsafety.gov/~fsg/fsgpath.html

Centers for Disease Control and Prevention
http://www.cdc.gov/ncidod/dbmd/diseaseinfo/foodborneinfections_g.htm

Cliver DO. Plastic and wooden cutting boards.
http://faculty.vetmed.ucdavis.edu/faculty/docliver/Research/cuttingboard.htm

FDA Center for Food Safety and Applied Nutrition. Gateway to government sources on food safety.
http://www.foodsafety.gov/

FDA Center for Food Safety and Applied Nutrition. Food Safety Facts for Microwave Ovens
http://www.foodsafety.gov/~fsg/fs-mwave.html

Fonseca JM, Ravishankar S. Safer salads. American Scientist. 95: 6 Pp: 494-501 Nov-Dec 2007.

North Carolina Department of Agriculture and Consumer Services. Bad bug book for kids.
http://www.agr.state.nc.us/cyber/kidswrld/foodsafe/badbug/badbug.htm

Plants For A Future (http://www.pfaf.org/index.php)

University of California, Davis. Statewide Integrated Pest Management Program. How to Manage Pests. Pests of Homes, Structures, People, and Pets. Pantry Pests
http://www.ipm.ucdavis.edu/PMG/PESTNOTES/pn7452.html#MANAGEMENT

USDA. Center for Food Safety and Applied Nutrition. Food Safety For YOU! Refrigerator & Freezer Storage Chart. http://www.cfsan.fda.gov/~dms/fttstore.html

USDA. Center for Food Safety and Applied Nutrition. Food Safety For YOU! The "411" On the 4 Cs! Clean, Cook, Combat Cross-Contamination, and Chill http://www.cfsan.fda.gov/~dms/ftt-411.html

USDA. Cutting boards and food safety. http://www.fsis.usda.gov/Fact_Sheets/Cutting_Boards_and_Food_Safety/index.asp

USDA Food Safety and Inspection Service. Washing Food: Does it Promote Food Safety? http://www.fsis.usda.gov/Fact_Sheets/Does_Washing_Food_Promote_Food_Safety/index.asp

USDA MyPyramid. Tips to help you eat fruits. http://www.mypyramid.gov/pyramid/fruits_tips.html

USDA. Food Safety and Inspection Service. Shell Eggs from Farm to Table. http://www.fsis.usda.gov/fact_sheets/Focus_On_Shell_Eggs/index.asp

Chapter Six

Mansfeld's World Database of Agricultural and Horticultural Crops. http://mansfeld.ipk-gatersleben.de/pls/htmldb_pgrc/f?p=185:3:3071540605148816::NO:::

US probiotics. http://www.usprobiotics.org/

Chapter Seven

USDA Directory of farmers markets. http://www.ams.usda.gov/farmersmarkets/

Directory and information on Community Supported Agriculture. http://www.localharvest.org/csa/

Research on canned food nutritional values: University of California, Davis Nutrition Comparison Study "Nutritional Comparison of Fresh, Frozen and Canned Fruits and Vegetables"
Part 1 http://www.mealtime.org/uploadedFiles/Mealtime/Content/jsfaarticle_partiucdavis_april07.pdf
Part 2 http://www.mealtime.org/uploadedFiles/Mealtime/Content/jsfaarticle_partiiucdavis_may07.pdf

Resource for recipes from the pantry using canned foods. http://www.mealtime.org/

University of Illinois Study "Nutrient Conservation in Canned, Frozen and Fresh Foods"
http://nutrican.fshn.uiuc.edu/
http://www.mealtime.org/uploadedFiles/Mealtime/Content/1997_nutrition_study_final.pdf

Chapter Eight

Danlac, Canada. Starter Cultures and Starter Culture Media http://www.danlac.com

National Center for Home Food Preservation. Fermented Foods: Kefir
http://www.uga.edu/nchfp/publications/nchfp/factsheets/kefir.html

National Center for Home Food Preservation. Fermenting Yogurt at Home
http://www.uga.edu/nchfp/publications/nchfp/factsheets/yogurt.html

University of Missouri Extension. Making Yogurt at Home: Country Living Series.
http://extension.missouri.edu/explore/hesguide/foodnut/gh1183.htm

University of Nebraska–Lincoln Extension. Making yogurt at home.
http://www.ianrpubs.unl.edu/epublic/pages/publicationD.jsp?publicationId=525

Chapter Nine

CDC, Fruits and veggies, more matters. http://www.fruitsandveggiesmatter.gov/month/index.html

EatingWell http://www.eatingwell.com/

Epicurious http://www.epicurious.com/recipesmenus/

Food Network http://www.foodnetwork.com/food/cooking/

FoodieView http://www.foodieview.com

National Honey Board http://www.honey.com/consumers/

Post Punk Kitchen http://www.theppk.com/recipes/

Recipezaar http://www.recipezaar.com/

Whole Foods Market: Produce http://www.wholefoodsmarket.com/products/produce.php

Chapter Ten

Abrahamsson TR, Jakobsson T, Böttcher MF, Fredrikson M, Jenmalm MC, Björkstén B, Oldaeus G. Probiotics in prevention of IgE-associated eczema: a double-blind, randomized, placebo-controlled trial. J Allergy Clin Immunol. 2007 May;119(5):1174-80.

Bakker-Zierikzee AM, Tol EA, Kroes H, Alles MS, Kok FJ, Bindels JG. Faecal SIgA secretion in infants fed on pre- or probiotic infant formula. Pediatr Allergy Immunol. 2006 Mar;17(2):134-40.

Binns CW, Lee AH, Harding H, Gracey M, Barclay DV. The CUPDAY Study: prebiotic-probiotic milk product in 1-3-year-old children attending childcare centres. Acta Paediatr. 2007 Nov;96(11):1646-50.

Caramia G, Atzei A, Fanos V. Probiotics and the skin. Clin Dermatol. 2008 Jan-Feb;26(1):4-11.

Corrêa NB, Péret Filho LA, Penna FJ, Lima FM, Nicoli JR. A randomized formula controlled trial of Bifidobacterium lactis and Streptococcus thermophilus for prevention of antibiotic-associated diarrhea in infants. J Clin Gastroenterol. 2005 May-Jun;39(5):385-9.

Costalos C, Kapiki A, Apostolou M, Papathoma E. The effect of a prebiotic supplemented formula on growth and stool microbiology of term infants. Early Hum Dev. 2008 Jan;84(1):45-9.

de Vrese M, Stegelmann B et al 2001. Probiotics-compensation for lactase insufficiency. Am. J Clin Nutr 73 (Suppl): 421S-429S.

Fukushima Y, Kawata Y, Hara H, Terada A, Mitsuoka T. Effect of a probiotic formula on intestinal immunoglobulin A production in healthy children. Int J Food Microbiol. 1998 Jun 30;42(1-2):39-44.

Hamilton-Miller JM. Probiotics and prebiotics in the elderly. Postgrad Med J. 2004 Aug;80(946):447-51.

Hickson M, D'Souza AL, Muthu N, Rogers TR, Want S, Rajkumar C, Bulpitt CJ.Use of probiotic Lactobacillus preparation to prevent diarrhoea associated with antibiotics: randomised double blind placebo controlled trial. BMJ. 2007 Jul 14;335(7610):80. Epub 2007 Jun 29.

Isolauri E, Arvola T, Sutas Y. Moilanen E, Salimen S. Probiotics in the management of atopic eczema. Clin. Exp Allergy 2000:30:1604-10.

Isolauri E. Dietary modification of atopic disease: Use of probiotics in the prevention of atopic dermatitis. Curr Allergy Asthma Rep. 2004 Jul;4(4):270-5.

Jakobsson T et al The effect of oral supplementation of Lactobacillus reuteri on the immunological composition of breast milk. Ped Gastroenterol Nutr 2005 40 (5):624, abstract OP 4-05

Kalliomäki M, Salminen S, Poussa T, Isolauri E. Probiotics during the first 7 years of life: a cumulative risk reduction of eczema in a randomized, placebo-controlled trial. J Allergy Clin Immunol. 2007 Apr;119(4):1019-21. Epub 2007 Feb 7.

Marteau P, Cuillerier E, Meance S, Gerhardt MF, Myara A, Bouvier M, Bouley C, Tondu F, Bommelaer G, Grimaud JC. Bifidobacterium animalis strain DN-173 010 shortens the colonic transit time in healthy women: a double-blind, randomized, controlled study. Aliment Pharmacol Ther. 2002 Mar;16(3):587-93.

MedlinePlus. Irritable bowel syndrome. http://www.nlm.nih.gov/medlineplus/irritablebowelsyndrome.html

Mohan R, Koebnick C, Schildt J, Schmidt S, Mueller M, Possner M, Radke M, Blaut M. Effects of Bifidobacterium lactis Bb12 supplementation on intestinal microbiota of preterm infants: a double-blind, placebo-controlled, randomized study. J Clin Microbiol. 2006 Nov;44(11):4025-31.

Moro G, Minoli I, Mosca M, Fanaro S, Jelinek J, Stahl B, Boehm G. Dosage-related bifidogenic effects of galacto- and fructooligosaccharides in formula-fed term infants. J Pediatr Gastroenterol Nutr. 2002 Mar;34(3):291-5.

Nestle Nutrition Institute. Probiotics: Implications for Pediatric Health. 2006

Nordstrom S. Pediatric Research 58:415 Occurrence of Lactobacillus reuteri, lactobacilli and Bifidobacteria in human breast milk. Referenced in: Nestle Nutrition Institute.

Probiotics: Implications for Pediatric Health. 2006.Palmer C, Bik EM, DiGiulio DB, Relman DA, Brown PO. Development of the Human Infant Intestinal Microbiota. PLoS Biology. Vol. 5, No. 7, e177 doi:10.1371/journal.pbio.0050177. http://biology.plosjournals.org/perlserv/?request=get-document&doi=10.1371/journal.pbio.0050177

Pietzak M. Presentation: "The use of probiotics in NEC and IBD" Advances in Perinatal Pediatric Nutrition July 16, 2007 Stanford University.

Probiotics. Med Lett Drugs Ther. 2007 Aug 13;49(1267):66-8.

Probiotics: Their Potential to Impact Human Health addresses the biological processes and physiological benefits of probiotics. CAST Issue Paper Number 36 October 2007. www.cast-science.org

Raloff, J. Nuturing our Microbes Science News vol 173 March 1, 2008 p138-139 www.sciencenews.org)

Reid G, Beuerman D, Heinemann C, Bruce AW. Probiotic Lactobacillus dose required to restore and maintain a normal vaginal flora. FEMS Immunol Med Microbiol. 2001 Dec;32(1):37-41.

Reuter G. The Lactobacillus and Bifidobacterium microflora of the human intestine: composition and succession. Curr Issues Intest Microbiol. 2001 Sep;2(2):43-53.

Saavedra JM, Abi-Hanna A, Moore N, Yolken RH. Long-term consumption of infant formulas containing live probiotic bacteria: tolerance and safety. Am J Clin Nutr. 2004 Feb;79(2):261-7.

Saavedra JM, Bauman NA, Oung I, Perman JA, Yolken RH. Feeding of Bifidobacterium bifidum and Streptococcus thermophilus to infants in hospital for prevention of diarrhoea and shedding of rotavirus. Lancet. 1994 Oct 15;344(8929):1046-9.

Salminen S, Isaulari E. Intestinal colonization, microbiota, and probiotics. (J Pediatr 2006;149:S115-S120)

Salminen S. Presentation; Intestinal Microbiota and Infant Health Advances in Perinatal Pediatric Nutrition July 16, 2007 Stanford University.

Savino F, Pelle E, Palumeri E, Oggero R, Miniero R. Lactobacillus reuteri (American Type Culture Collection Strain 55730) versus simethicone in the treatment of infantile colic: a prospective randomized study. Pediatrics. 2007 Jan;119(1):e124-30.

Sazawal S, Dhingra U, et al. Efficacy of milk fortified with a probiotic. IN: Nestle Nutrition Institute. Probiotics: Implications for Pediatric Health. 2006

Szajewska H, Setty M, Mrukowicz J, Guandalini S. Probiotics in gastrointestinal diseases in children: hard and not-so-hard evidence of efficacy. J Pediatr Gastroenterol Nutr. 2006 May;42(5):454-75.

Trenev, Natasha. Probiotics: Nature's Internal Healers. New York: Avery, 1998.

Veereman G. Pediatric applications of inulin and oligofructose. J Nutr. 2007 Nov;137(11 Suppl):2585S-2589S.

Weizman Z, Asli G, Alsheikh A. Effect of a probiotic infant formula on infections in child care centers: comparison of two probiotic agents. Pediatrics. 2005 Jan;115(1):5-9.

Whorwell PJ, Altringer L, Morel J, Bond Y, Charbonneau D, O'Mahony L, Kiely B, Shanahan F, Quigley EM. Efficacy of an encapsulated probiotic Bifidobacterium infantis 35624 in women with irritable bowel syndrome. Am J Gastroenterol. 2006 Jul;101(7):1581-90.

Ziegler E, Vanderhoof JA, Petschow B, Mitmesser SH, Stolz SI, Harris CL, Berseth CL. Term infants fed formula supplemented with selected blends of prebiotics grow normally and have soft stools similar to those reported for breast-fed infants. J Pediatr Gastroenterol Nutr. 2007 Mar;44(3):359-64.

www.ingramcontent.com/pod-product-compliance
Lightning Source LLC
Chambersburg PA
CBHW081156270326

41930CB00014B/3178